AN UNHOLY TRINITY

ABOUT THE AUTHOR

Liam Kirwan is currently Professor of Surgery, Penang Medical College, Malaysia. Prior to that he worked for 35 years as a Consultant/Professor in a large public hospital in the Irish Health Service, where he served on innumerable administrative bodies and committees at both local and national level. Liam has worked in surgery in Ireland, Great Britain, the United States and now Malaysia, and has extensive experience of their diverse healthcare systems. He is the author of 120 scientific papers as well as a previous book, *Political Correctness and the Surgeon.*

AN UNHOLY TRINITY

Medicine, Politics and Religion in Ireland

Liam Kirwan

The Liffey Press

Published by
The Liffey Press Ltd
Raheny Shopping Centre, Second Floor
Raheny, Dublin 5, Ireland
www.theliffeypress.com

A catalogue record of this book is
available from the British Library.

ISBN 978-1-908308-92-4

Printed in Ireland by SprintPrint.

CONTENTS

Preface

There are few things as important to a country as the standard of healthcare that is available to its citizens. This standard is measured by two parameters, quality and access. It is generally agreed that, in Ireland, the quality is excellent but the access at the time of writing is deplorable. Successive governments, of whatever ideology, have acquiesced in this inequitable access to services.

The genesis of the present Irish Health Service has been extensively documented but mainly by historians, administrators and journalists – an ingredient is lacking. Doctors working within it have written little that is definitive on the structure of the service. In particular, the medical profession, engaged in what is in effect a frozen conflict with the Department of Health, has indulged in little critical self-analysis.

The events of 1950, when Church and medicine conspired together to destroy a Minister for Health of independent mind, Noël Browne, laid the foundations for the present dysfunction. While the history of those events is well documented, there is a tendency to forget. Furthermore, only those who work day to day within the service, and acquaint themselves with its history, can trace the current deficiencies to watershed events in the past.

In an effort to combine my medical (surgical) insights with those who have written about Irish history generally, and about medical administration in particular, I have drawn on many notable works. The work of Ruth Barrington is definitive in this regard, up to 1970, as is that of Brendan Hensey – both from the administrative perspective. Historians also have included in their broader works sections which have been informative in this regard. These include Ronan Fanning and John Whyte. Of particular relevance to the subject addressed here are the works of later writers of biographies of characters whose actions were fundamental to where the Irish Health Service finds itself today. These are John Cooney (John Charles McQuaid), David McCullagh (John A. Costello) and John Horgan (Noël Browne). Finally, the belated (1986) autobiography of Noël Browne himself chimes with much that the author has observed over the years.

I would like to express my appreciation to the staff of the following archival institutions: National Archives of Ireland, Dublin Diocesan Archives, Cork City and County Archives and University College Cork Archives.

My thanks to Kiran Shandu for adroitly turning my idea for a suitable image into a lovely cover design.

I am grateful to Barry Ferris whose penetrating observations from an early stage were extremely constructive. Fergus Shanahan offered encouragement when it was much needed. Maurice Manning read it when it had many faults and I thank him. Finally, my wife Marie, always encouraging, by trenchant observation and criticism instilled a rigour which I might not otherwise have been able to achieve.

This book is not the work of a professional historian; others do that better. It does, however, attempt, from insights gleaned on the inside over a lifetime, to find in history the seeds of where Irish medicine is now and to trace those seeds through to the inequities of today.

Liam Kirwan
October 2016

Notable Quotations

'That the executive committee appoint a Propaganda Sub-Committee with a view to educating the public as to the dangers of a State Medical Service'. *Decision of the Irish Medical Association Central Council, December 1950, circulated to members.*

'The Cancer of Socialised Medicine'. *Irish Medical Association Proposals for a Voluntary Contributory State-Aided Medical Scheme, 1951.*

'In my opinion the establishment of Vocational Schools and the Health Act are the two greatest blows which Catholic social principles have received in this country'. *Alfred O'Rahilly, President of University College Cork, letter to Archbishop McQuaid, 1954.*

'We regard with the greatest apprehension the proposal to give local medical officers the right to tell Catholic girls and women how they should behave in regard to this sphere of conduct at once so delicate and sacred'. *Letter from the Bishop of Ferns, on behalf of the Hierarchy, to the Taoiseach, 1950.*

'Doctors trained in institutions in which we have no confidence may be appointed as medical officers'. *Letter from the Bishop of Ferns, on behalf of the Hierarchy, to the Taoiseach, 1950.*

'It is for the Hierarchy alone to say whether or no the scheme contained anything contrary to Catholic moral teaching'. *Letter from Taoiseach to Noël Browne, Minister for Health, regarding the Mother and Child scheme, 1951*

'As a Catholic I accept the rulings of Their Lordships the Hierarchy without question'. *Noël Browne in his resignation statement, 1951.*

'Transfer of hospitals to the Minister'. *Enabling clause in British National Health Service Act, 1946.*

'The allowance is a private contractual arrangement between the Board and the Chief Executive.... On that basis, Our Lady's Children's Hospital Crumlin will not be making any public comment on the salary details of the private contract'. *Statement by publicly funded Our Lady's Hospital regarding its accountability on executive pay, 2013.*

To Marie

INTRODUCTION

The interface between politics and medicine is fascinating, varies considerably between different cultures and countries and is often fraught with friction between the two camps. The politician, having to submit himself to the caprice of the electorate, takes the pragmatic view that his first, and alas occasionally only, duty is to get elected. This disarmingly frank approach is singularly lacking in pomp. The doctor, however, particularly if he is of such tendency as to aspire to a leadership role in his profession, is not always bereft of such pomp. Indeed, he or she may irritate their political masters by seeking to cloak what the politician sees as hubris, in layers of Hippocratic justification. The medical man, or woman, would do well, however, to realise that Hippocrates is little known in the parliamentary constituency, and less again does he inhabit the mind of he who must practice 'the art of the possible'.[1] This latter exponent of 'the possible' knows that ideals are expensive and has come to realise that Hippocratic ones, as a result of scientific advances in medicine, are catastrophically so in the modern world. And yet there are great votes in 'health'.

The word 'health' is embedded in a visceral way in many languages. In the twentieth century Ireland of this observer's youth, use of the word health was ubiquitous most particularly in the daily parlance of the less fortunate who, living closer to the edge, were in greater danger of losing it. This was particularly so in the countryside, where traditional modes of

1

expression, not perceived as a badge of unsophistication as in the city, held sway. Indeed, this mode of expression lingered even in the urban cognoscenti who could, if required, remove themselves to Switzerland to heal their tubercular cavities. Even the well-off were still vulnerable to a multitude of other contagions and afflictions impervious to their money, and had in their aspirations occasional resort to the word 'health' as a concession to their vulnerability and in the hope of staving off dissolution.

The formerly commonplace greeting 'may the Lord spare you your health' is now rarely heard. The Lord, of course, is much out of favour in Ireland and as a consequence is now excused this national responsibility. Thus health catastrophes, which formerly were accepted as 'the will of God', are now frequently attributed to the delinquency of the State or its agents. Replacing God in this responsibility is no small challenge and is fraught with much risk for the politician, but, in the event of success, promises even more spectacular electoral reward.

Thus the politician, motivated by the abundance of votes so to be garnered, has stepped into the breach vacated by God.

It is not surprising that this departure should, on occasion, have drawn politicians, in their exercise of temporal authority, into conflict with those who exercised authority of the spiritual kind, Their Lordships the Bishops. The Church, after all, had been the main provider of and owned healthcare (such as it was) in many European countries since the Middle Ages and was jealous of its prerogatives. Furthermore, medicine in that tradition, which was much to the benefit of church prestige, was dispensed as largesse or charity, rather than as a right. Although many European Church establishments had yielded to state intrusion into medicine, nowhere had the Bishops held on to their prerogatives in this regard with more tenacity than in the Ireland of mid-twentieth century. It thus became inevitable that the intrusion of vulgar politicians upon their pious prerogatives would rouse Their Episcopal Lordships to action. This was particularly so given the Episcopal personalities involved in mid-twentieth century Ireland, spectacularly spared as they were of any democratic pretension.

The word 'vulgar' as used here is one of approbation rather than condescension and connotes the politician's democratic connection to the common people. The politician collects not tithes,[2] but taxes. The collectors of tithes, the clergy, could afford to be cavalier about the physical wellbeing of donors, concentrating instead on their spiritual welfare, the latter, of course, being much cheaper. The collectors of taxes, however, the politicians, are required to be more circumspect as a result of the necessity to subject themselves to the repeated tiresome intrusions of the ballot box.

The politician, because he is elected, carries great credibility with those who are innately democratic, and it is a redeeming feature of the human race that most, but not all,[3] can be so described. The political classes, however, were slow enough off the healthcare mark and in some instances, notably in the United States, Government involvement in healthcare is regarded by the right wing as the purest anathema. At the time of writing, 'Obamacare'[4] is under sustained attack by conservatives and it is not clear that the programme will be allowed to achieve its full potential in improving the lot of the most miserable. Societies where the poor are allowed to be so neglected are characterised by a large impoverished, poorly educated, disenfranchised rump. Advocates of 'Small Government'[5] can in such environments, and with some perversity, advance the argument that the government has no business in healthcare and that the taxpayer should not be so burdened.

In this American 'Small Government' culture a strange inversion takes place. The aspiring politician, who advocates strong Government healthcare interventions for the people, is as likely, contrary to all European intuition, to be rebuffed as to be rewarded at the ballot box (or the electronic polling booth). In this model of democracy, which indeed the right wing in America considers suitable for export to other countries, by use of force if necessary, the inconvenient impoverished rump is deleted from the consciousness of the comfortable.

It is interesting to note that, in the promulgation of this conservative ideology in America, in healthcare as in much else, right wing religious elements have been to the fore. This is relevant to the manner in which healthcare infrastructure has evolved in Ireland. The tripartite relationship between medicine, politics and religion, and particularly the former and the latter, has often been excessively intimate and did, in large measure, determine the dubious structure of the health service which the country has inherited. This structure had embedded in it the ingredients for the dysfunction which has increasingly manifested itself with the passage of time. Dysfunction is maximal in times of economic stress and bears most heavily on the weakest citizens. This *ménage* à *trois* did not always act in the interest of all the citizens.

Early attempts to provide a measure of healthcare for the less fortunate came mainly from institutional religion and were motivated by genuine and admirable charity. Government regimes in many countries, mostly not elected by universal suffrage, while professing paternalism, were excused the sanction of the ballot box and saw little benefit in concerning themselves with the health of the citizen. Indeed the concept of *le citoyen* emerging from the French Revolution was less than comfortable for such regimes who felt that the genie belonged in the bottle.

The real genie however was scientific medicine released from the bottle by the prepared minds of Louis Pasteur,[6] Joseph Lister,[7] Ignaz Semmelweis,[8] Robert Koch[9] and many others. Theretofore, the fashionable physician had been distinguished by his sartorial elegance and his mastery of the classics. It is not, of course, that such attributes are without attraction, but rather that their exponents had a regrettable tendency to lapse into hocus pocus which was a poor match for the emerging scientific method.[10] The evidence-based scientific method will debunk hocus pocus every time if given a fair hearing, but its practitioner may find himself unloved by entrenched powerful elements. Such elements may be medical or religious or, more menacingly, an alliance of the two.

In any case, following the release of the Pasteur genie, and the discoveries stemming therefrom, it became possible for doctors to do things more meaningful than drain pus, apply poultices and spout Latin. More hospitals appeared and became the focus of expanded activity which, in those early days, was largely of a surgical nature.

1

BEGINNINGS

The nascent institutional interest in medicine in Ireland first manifested itself in the shape of the Charitable Infirmary.[11] Such early institutions, in the eighteenth century, were secular and were truly charitable by name and charitable by nature, and depended on donations from the moneyed classes. Scientific medicine had not yet arrived and the charitable institutions were mainly places of care and maintenance rather than of medical intervention as it is known today. The elected politician, increasingly the norm rather than the exception, was gradually drawn into the administration of such places although he did not yet have at his disposal, for disbursement, significant public monies as he has today. It was, nevertheless, no electoral disadvantage to be ensconced on the board of the local Charitable Infirmary. Funding, however, was prised out of the propertied classes, in the nineteenth century and subsequently, only with the greatest of difficulty and such institutions, always strapped for cash, afforded to the lower orders of society only a basic level of service.

At the outset it should be stated without equivocation that the contribution of religious orders of nuns and voluntary Christian effort generally, to the early development of hospital services in Ireland, and indeed in many places throughout the world, was heroic. The nuns embraced with energy and determination the now discarded 'Nightingale' tradition.

Curiously, however, this epochal contribution to medicine, education and much else for more than a century has been, in a historicide born out of political correctness, almost deleted from the national consciousness. Eaten bread is soon forgotten.

As the twentieth century advanced 'charitable' institutions, now increasingly referred to as 'Voluntary Hospitals', began to derive more of their income from public rather than charitable sources. In parallel the Catholic Church, its prestige greatly enhanced earlier by the adherence of its rank and file clergy to the people during the famine and by able leadership,[12] had developed its own hospitals[13] vested in various orders of Religious but ruled by the Bishops with a rod of iron.

Even in those hospitals which the Church did not own, the Bishops vicariously exercised control by inserting nuns, constrained by vows of obedience. This insertion of nuns enabled the Church, in the manner in which imperial governments sent a gunboat, to project power from a distance and at little cost. By the time mid-twentieth century arrived the dominant Church, either directly or vicariously, controlled almost the entire hospital infrastructure of the country. The upshot of this trend was that, by the time under discussion, medicine and a great deal besides was controlled by the Church of Rome to such an extent that the Republic, declared with bullets in 1916 and formalised with bombast in 1948,[14] had degenerated into a theocracy.

These 'gunboat' nuns deployed in this way were all well and good as far as it went in institutions designed mainly for the less fortunate. It quickly became apparent, however, that a better class of place was required for the ruling orders; a place more conducive to their comfort and dignity. A word of caution is appropriate with regard to our use of the somewhat *risqué* term 'ruling orders'. We are not referring here just to aristocracy, landed gentry or captains of industry, but also to the upwardly mobile adherents to the majority religion, now more numerous, more prosperous and with increased ambition, and pretension in proportion. It is also relevant to what is about to happen that, as a result of the prestige of having a priest in the family and the talent thus recruited, organised religion is, to a considerable degree, controlled at this time by the scions of such upwardly mobile families.

And so to the arrangement contrived by the better heeled and their spiritual elite for their medical repair when afflicted – the freestanding totally private hospital. Now, it should be clearly stated at the outset that there is nothing wrong with this *per se*. The matter is, alas, not so straightforward a moral or indeed political issue as it might seem at first sight.

Such private medical institutions, with a few exceptions Catholic and Church-owned, were designated as charities as indeed would have been normal in many other countries. They were, furthermore, performing the same corporal works of mercy as publicly funded institutions catering for the less opulent. This, however, on occasion resulted in the enigmatic situation of two 'charitable' institutions quite close together physically but poles apart with regard to the economic status and social station of their clientele. The definition of charity, as applied to medicine, was becoming elasticated.

Charity is generally defined as 'devoted to the assistance of those in need'. According to the early Christian concept from which the word derives,[15] charity meant caring – giving to the poor. This is well exemplified by the biblical story of Dives and Lazarus,[16] a narrative on which generations of Irish children had been weaned. The rich and self-indulgent Dives is cautioned by St Luke that he should, towards the purpose of his salvation, be charitable towards the starving and disease-ridden Lazarus.

The concept of charity for the poor is innately noble and edifying. It is universally understood and places no strain on the imagination. Poverty and charity are birds of a feather and, after all, 'the poor are always with us'.[17] There is, however, a flaw.

Without wishing to be churlish towards the great Evangelist, it is nevertheless difficult to banish the thought that this latter quotation does little service to the less fortunate and tends rather to normalise their plight. Since their presence is thus deemed inevitable, and by so formidable an authority, it is nobody's fault and the more fortunate may therefore, without fear of damnation, remove themselves to more salubrious quarters for their medical treatment and much else.

It is to the credit of the Catholic Church that it had sought, through its institutions, to take medical care of its flock over the full span of the socio-economic spectrum. It is less reassuring, however, that the Church was easily able to countenance, even at this early stage, the triage of patients according to their means rather than their pathology and medical need. It was and is, of course, perfectly reasonable that patients should triage themselves towards comfort and a better healthcare environment – at their own expense. But was the Church deviating from its true path by so exerting itself on behalf of Dives while Lazarus was in such a wretched condition and in much greater need? It would be many years before Pope Francis called for a reorientation towards what he called 'a poor Church'. In the meantime, however, the Church has given its imprimatur to separation and to a duality of standards which has endured, to the disgruntlement of many.

The private Church-owned hospitals which thus sprung up, and indeed the private annexes of otherwise public or charitable institutions, were staffed largely by nuns, then abundant. These had great credibility. They had taken vows of poverty which in those days were enforced, on the individual if not on the institution, with an iron discipline. The irony of those sworn to poverty being deployed to pamper the rich was apparent to few. The nuns had also taken vows of obedience – total obedience to the whims and diktats of the local Bishops. The Bishops were laying down the template for the future hybrid (later to be known as 'two tier') system and they were using the benevolence of the nuns to do so.

Strangely the absence of Lazarus from the halls and wards of the new private rich charitable places, whose denizens live by the Gospels, including presumably that of St Luke, passes unnoticed without a hint of irony. The comfortable classes and their spiritual leaders, drawn from the same echelon of society, have redefined charity and, as is well known, charity begins at home. The die of self-deception was cast.

Such nun-run private institutions would surely have been the envy of any modern day hospital manager. All the woes that beset him today were in the distant future. Spared the tedium of democracy, hiring and firing was by whim: a system heavily reliant on suitability rather than the altogether less predictable criterion of merit. Catholic orthodoxy was *de rigueur*. Indeed, the Bishops, either personally or through formidable matriarchal nuns, kept a tight rein on appointments to all senior positions.

Meanwhile the politician, while to his credit discharging his responsibility, spotted an opportunity. While the Bishops might affect concern for the immortal souls of their flock, the politician concerned himself with the altogether less nebulous matter of their votes. Few things are as conducive to the harvesting of votes as the provision of free healthcare and thus was the politician sucked in. Many times since, indeed, has he cursed this populist departure and attempted to extricate himself from the fiscal nightmare. There are, however, as we have observed 'great votes in health', and any attempt at retrenchment in times of revenue fatigue can result in that greatest of all catastrophes, electoral oblivion.

Thus did the politician become a prisoner of the healthcare treadmill.

The designation of an institution or activity as charitable for tax purposes is a matter of the law[18] and of Government policy and, in twentieth century Ireland, the makers of that policy were joined at the hip with the Catholic Bishops.

The politician – and it is he after all who levies taxes – prompted by the bosses of organised religion, determine that institutions dispensing rich charity, although profitable, should be exempted from the rigours of supporting the public purse. The business formula was perfect: abundant cheap labour, vows of obedience in the imposition of which fear of hell was an invaluable asset, and a warm feeling of piety sustained by the convenient belief – the absence of Lazarus notwithstanding – that the mission was a charitable one. All of this had the advantages for the moneyed classes of keeping comfort up and price down. It was also encouraging those who could pay, to separate themselves from those who could not, for their medical care – two tiers.

And so it continued for generations, but nothing lasts forever.

2

Equilibrium Disturbed

Great upheavals in the affairs of the world have an unhappy way of upsetting comfortable equilibrium. Citizens who get a glimpse of something better may no longer wish to endure that which, theretofore, they had considered inevitable. Thus in the aftermath of World War II, while medical science was jolted forward by the experience of managing military trauma so also social science and consciousness was likewise aroused, as by all great upheavals. The upshot was that the masses, particularly in Great Britain from which Ireland was nominally detached but intimately bound, demanded a more equitable slice of the cake and of the health cake in particular. They did not want the crumbs from the table of Dives anymore. They did not want the poor charity anymore. They wanted the real thing, a properly organised health service, as of right.

The British politician and the ruling caste, in the aftermath of the war, canny to the shifting equilibrium and altered social expectation, were obliged, in the interest of their preservation, to trim their sails to the new wind. They were moved in this direction by the tedious fact that in a parliamentary democracy, Dives and Lazarus weigh in equally at the ballot box. Indeed, it was at this time a feature of Irish life that Lazarus, because of the nation's history of struggle, put great store on the exercise of his franchise and rarely failed to turn out on polling day.

The new wind to which the British politician and indeed those in many other places were trimming their sails took a while to arrive in Ireland. With regard to ideological orientations left and right, the population was not politically savvy. Indeed, anything vaguely to the left of centre was viewed as the work of the devil. This suspicion was fuelled by the all powerful Catholic Church and its 'political Bishops'.[19] Chief among these was God's main man in Ireland, the extremely able, autocratic and ultra-conservative Archbishop of Dublin, His Grace Dr John Charles McQuaid.

Many Young Men of Twenty

In the aftermath of World War II Ireland was in an economic time warp. Having embraced neutrality in the conflict – a rather misty Celtic neutrality which was decidedly biased towards the Allies[20] and which incarcerated German servicemen who were cast upon our shores, but allowed many downed British airmen quietly to repatriate themselves by crossing the border into Northern Ireland – economic oblivion followed. There was no post-war reconstruction boom because there had been no war destruction. Closely tied economically and historically to its victorious neighbour, whose attitude was epitomised by the virulent hostility of Beaverbrook Newspapers, Ireland was left to its fate. The role of the Irish was (reminiscent of the earlier Cromwellian sentence, to be 'hewers of wood and drawers of water') to be providers of cheap food and strong backed emigrant labour to John Bull's main island.

And it was to the neighbouring island that the life blood of economy the young and mostly healthy flowed. The stereotypical Irish immigrant was the carrier of the hod.[21] He had not made 'his body a weapon of the war'[22] but its broad and poorly educated shoulders were ideal fodder for the reconstruction. It should be said that he was reasonably received and well paid by his hosts. The country of his birth, however, he being of the legion of the Lazarites, confined his pre-emigration conditioning to that overwhelming preoccupation of the time, his spiritual welfare. The 'many young men of twenty'[23] who said goodbye would be alright as long as they did not 'eat black puddings on a Friday'.

'THE NATIONAL HEALTH'

Strangely, the many young men of twenty found, on their arrival in England, that while their immortal souls were in dire jeopardy, their equally perishable bodies were generously catered for by a new system increasingly mentioned in dispatches home as the National Health Service. Furthermore, since young men are little encumbered by Faustian nightmares, they had little difficulty in forsaking idleness, poverty and depression at home for jobs, money and accessible medical care in England. They opted to forsake the certainty of salvation in Catholic Ireland for the compensations of 'Pagan England' – an expression much in vogue at the time – and to take their chances with the devil later.

And it was not only the 'young men of twenty' who went. While economic stagnation was stultifying for the male it was doubly so for the female and the spirited ones got out in great numbers. Instead of, as in previous generations, being condemned to the drudgery of 'service' (in the big house) they were avidly recruited to nurse training in the burgeoning new National Health Service (1948) and were highly valued. They sniffed out this form of education – always the holy grail of the Irish peasant – which, and this almost defied comprehension, was provided free by a society and a government which they had been conditioned to view with suspicion. These young women were often from the less well connected levels of Irish society. Access to such nursing education in their own country, in leading hospitals mostly controlled by the Church and where they would have had to pay for their tuition, was denied them in favour of young ladies from the business, professional or strong farmer class who would of course be deemed more 'suitable'.

As a result of this migration and the consequent letters home, the strangest reports concerning the folly and profligacy of this new creature the 'National Health' began to reach our shores.

It was reported that, as a matter of right, everything was provided free under the 'National Health' – even to Irish immigrants. Spectacles, admittedly of rather rudimentary appearance evocative of 'Orphan Annie'[24] but later made fashionable by Beatle John Lennon, were tested for and handed out with abandon. The dispensing of free false teeth to the masses struck a particular chord in an Ireland long known for its diabolical dentition. In a place where the most that could be expected by the masses, and this indeed at their own expense, was the pulling of teeth that were painful and rotten, reports of full conservative dentistry provided *gratis* stretched to its limit what modest level of credulity the average Irish peasant, or indeed his more gentrified urban cousin, could muster. Clearly the veracity of such reports had to be put to the test and the native cunning of a race still in or only lately removed from the countryside was not found wanting.

Decades before the phenomenon would be crystallised in words, medical tourism was born.

And so it came to pass that many a mother whose daughter was 'nursing in England' went to visit her and came back with a fine new set of dentures the equal of those sported by her betters at great expense, and all provided by the bounty of His Majesty's Government, now viewed with a less jaundiced eye by these opportunist beneficiaries from his former other island.

In describing the munificence of Perfidious Albion[25] and her National Health Service to the casually visiting poorly sighted, edentulous and indeed those afflicted in many other parts, a peculiar quirk of language was brought to bear: the word 'service' was deleted from the end. This despised word had connoted in Ireland drudgery in 'the big house', or for many an Irish emigrant girl indentured service in Manhattan or Philadelphia. To be 'in service' was to be at the butt end and the stigmatised word had no place in describing the joyous tidings of largesse arriving daily form the other island. Thus, pending the arrival of national self-assurance, the word 'service' would be dispensed with and in the Irish countryside they would speak, with awe, only of the 'National Health'.

This was a time of national atrophy in Ireland.

The dispatches arriving from the 'National Health', in proportion to the scale of the emigration,[26] increased to a torrent. Hospitals were free. Surgery was free. The general practitioner was free. Maternity was free. There was in addition an incomprehensible array of payments, allowances, services and perks – all free.

Milk was given out free by the 'National Health' to schools and families. This enigma was, in an Ireland awash with milk and where rickets[27] was still rife, viewed as in no way ironic and did not occasion the least introspection; in fact, the contrary began to happen.

Soon reports began to appear questioning the wisdom of the State dispensing such largesse to its citizens. The innuendo was that it was fine for England to engage in such folly if she so wished, but Ireland knew better. Would such mollycoddling not be erosive of national self-reliance and moral fibre? Would the state not be drawn into places – private places – where it had no business to be? Would this not impose an intolerable burden upon the taxpayer? Foremost in articulating such conservative thoughts was the oracle of the Catholic Church, Archbishop McQuaid, who had a most incongruous (and indeed un-Christian) anxiety that the taxpayer should not be so burdened and, as evidence of this, we shall amply quote him *verbatim* later.

It should be noted that this was at a time when rural electrification had scarcely penetrated the hinterland, when

Bishops railed against 'the evils of mixed bathing'[28] and when, on occasion, the most riveting item on the main news bulletin from the national broadcaster was that the Pope had moved to his summer residence at Castelgandolfo.

LETTERS FROM AMERICA

In their Atlantic island the Irish occupy an entirely singular place geographically, historically, culturally and psychologically. Although visible in part from the British mainland, Ireland is psychologically in many other respects fixed in mid-Atlantic. It is not surprising that a nation, having endured almost a millennium of foreign domination, should seek to distance itself from its erstwhile oppressor. This mid-Atlantic fixation took its roots in a huge vociferous, politically savvy and upwardly mobile American diaspora.

The American diaspora also wrote home.

Letters from America reported on a nation which took a diametrically opposing approach to the provision of healthcare from that of the British National Health Service. Admittedly, there had been Franklin Roosevelt's 'New Deal', but that intervention had been undertaken only in order to resuscitate the economy from the great depression and confined itself to such matters as social security and public health. Indeed, conservative elements considered that these modest interventions were diabolical instruments and would be erosive of the self-reliance so treasured in the American Republic.

In America, the citizen, far from being mollycoddled, was required to make provision for his own healthcare privately. The concept of a comprehensive public scheme was anathema and, at a time when the cold war was ramping up, carried the taint of communism. In the land of opportunity – public bad, private good. There would be no American National Health Service; indeed, how alien these four words look on paper. The greatest curiosity exercising American doctors visiting Ireland for conferences then and for many years thereafter was not a scientific one but rather whether we had 'socialised medicine over here'. The credo was that of the *laissez faire*. In the land of the free you would have to pay dearly for your medicine.

And so it was reported in letters home.

Letters from America, although conjuring up conflicting emotions of joy and sadness, were exotic: they symbolised the colour of that place. The flimsy paper, the red and blue margin, the airmail sticker, the senders address for all to see, the fascinating stamps in metric currency, all excited the imagination as to the wonderful place whence they had come. Strewn out for sorting on the Post Office counter along with more mundane missives, they stuck out a mile. Their significance was appreciated by the country postman, who although heavily burdened particularly at Christmas and pedalling his laden bicycle into the December wind, delivered them with good humour to the door.

In a land of large families – then grown mainly for export – many a mother had offspring dispersed both to the United States and to England. Of course, reports arriving from eastern and western diaspora differed greatly and often described situations and attitudes which were polar opposites. The plenty of America was in stark contrast to the paucity and indeed the lingering post-war rationing of England. Likewise, the hyperbole and lack of inhibition of the New World was in marked contrast to the understatement and reserve of the old. Remarkably different also was the instinctive muting of one's Irishness in the land of the stereotyped hod carrier, as distinct from its open flaunting in America. For many a family whose young men of twenty had gone both east and west, these contrasting societal approaches were a cause of bemusement. The glamour of America was neutered by its remoteness, while the austerity of England was softened by its proximity.

But of all the differences reported from the two great foreign countries one stood out above all the others. In England they had the 'National Health'.

It is, of course, axiomatic that emigration is resorted to predominantly by the young and healthy. This latter description is, however, applied with some licence to the Irish population of mid-twentieth century. Infectious diseases, notably tuberculosis[29] and poliomyelitis,[30] were not controlled. Remarkably, England accepted all comers from Ireland without scrutiny – it was simply a matter of getting on 'the boat'. And off the boat came much pathology to be magnanimously assumed into the National Health Service where careful doctors had uppermost in their minds in dealing with the Irish (as they had with Asians later) a diagnosis of tuberculosis in its many and varied forms.

Uncle Sam, however, was having no truck with such foolishness. He was in business for profit not charity. He had replaced the spontaneity of Ellis Island with a panoply of screening procedures designed to deliver only the healthy and the productive. Uncle Sam had always done it his way and if you did not like it you could lump it. If you did not on arrival present him with evidence of full immunisation, negative serology and a clear chest x-ray to stick up on the viewing box right there, lump it you could.

The Irish citizen viewing such alternatives (the American versus the British) in medical provision through the limited prism of letters home, state-controlled radio and a heavily censored cinema, could see attractions in both.

MEDICINE AND THE CINEMA

In the cinema in particular, American medicine was always portrayed as glamorous, scientific and modern. Patients seemed always to be in perfect private rooms and were invariably happy, positive and respectful. Doctors enjoyed a reverence which to the outside sceptic appeared somewhat excessive and more than occasionally bordered on the unctuous. Nurses were uniformed to military standard, formidable and not to be trifled with. A difficulty with such cinematic portrayals, however, was that it was never made clear as to which segment or percentage of the population, or at what cost, such glamorous services were made available. Only the discerning would have noticed that Lazarus was rarely in the bed.

The hospital accountant did not star in such movies.

In the land of the 'National Health' British cinema was also hyperactive at this time. Towards the purpose of alleviating the tedium of post-war austerity, the cinema was pressed into frantic service. The output however was laced with a sexual innuendo and a vulgarity which contrasted starkly with the primness and propriety of American productions. The British cinematic approach to portraying medicine was entirely different and altogether less reverential to the establishment, i.e. the doctors. Prurience replaced primness and satire replaced respect. Comedy was generally the idiom. The set of the drama was not the private hospital room as in America, but the very public Nightingale ward. The dialogue was that of the working man and woman. The place appeared to be inhabited by real and earthy people rather than the more sanitised types portrayed in the American hospital.

Senior doctors in the British cinema's portrayal of the medical environment were cut down to size by satire and were indeed on occasion portrayed as buffoons.[31] Senior nurses, caricatured as the Matron were, it is true, portrayed as formidable, but her minions were trivialised and measured more by their endowment than their usefulness. It was with much misgiving that many an Irish mother sent her daughter into such an environment for nurse education, but the logistics and sense of loss were less than those occasioned by departure to America.

In mid-Atlantic theocratic Ireland, where there was a grand alliance between senior doctors and the Princes of the Church – always with a watchful eye to Castelgandolfo – the American approach chimed better.

CONFLICTING REPORTS

The 'National Health' however aroused great curiosity in Ireland and the people began to hope that the contagion would spread westward to benefit themselves. Also, there was in place in the Custom House[32] a left-leaning Minister for Health, Dr Noël Browne, known to be an admirer of the British service.

And all the while the reports came back: everything was free under the 'National Health.'

Reports from America ran quite to the contrary. All medical services there had to be paid for and paid for, by all accounts, through the nose. Common medical or surgical procedures were expensive beyond manageable levels of arithmetic. Medical emergencies of even intermediate severity could have a ruinous effect on family finances. True, the concept of medical insurance – scarcely known in Ireland – was embedded in the American psyche, but such insurance schemes were run by huge corporations for profit. American medicine was highly ideological and was conceived as an industry. The British National Health Service was no less ideological but was conceived, as is implicit in its naming, as a service with a large component of societal responsibility.

Thus by mid-twentieth century the ideological lines in Ireland were clearly drawn between those supporting two extremely diverse systems of healthcare provision. In the blue corner, with their creed of self-reliance and devil take the hindmost, were the Episcopal and medical advocates of the American way. In the appropriately named red corner, much admiring of the British National Health Service, were predictable elements of the left, but now, to the consternation of their adversaries, they included no less a personage than the Minister for Health, Dr Noël Browne.

Browne proposed a new Mother and Child Health Service to be made available during pregnancy, through delivery and its aftermath to cover all children up to the age of 16 years. To the great discomfiture of the leaders of medicine, he announced with some flamboyance that the service would be entirely free – there would be no means test. He made much of the fact that the patients would not have to pay the doctors. His proposal to nudge the health service in the direction of increased free public provision did not chime with the medical establishment.

America, greatly admired in Ireland, had emerged from the recent war victorious and vibrant. Its industry and technology, by its quality and depth, had swept the board. It felt assured that its system of government, based on Jeffersonian principles, was unsurpassed and was suitable for export. The remainder of the twentieth century and beyond would be American. This was all attributed to the benefits of unbridled capitalism and freebooting enterprise, which would apply to medicine as to all else. The received wisdom was that medicine would work best when run as a business and provided for a profit. It is not surprising that the American plutocracy, business and medical, should be comfortable with this analysis. However, non-metropolitan Americans on the middle and indeed lower rungs of the economic ladder, or not on it at all, many of whom would have benefited greatly from better publicly provided health services, were equally gulled into believing that the provision of such services, or 'socialised medicine' as it was stigmatised, would be the work of the devil himself.

The Irish Catholic Hierarchy of the time were of like mind and stigmatised the effort of the Minister for Health to provide free universal maternity and child services under his proposed Mother and Child Scheme as 'a costly bureaucratic scheme of nationalised medical service'.[33]

THE COMMUNIST BOGEYMAN

It is fair to acknowledge, since all things should be considered in their temporal context, that the great bogeyman of the time was communism. Josef Stalin, so recently an ally in the defeat of Hitler and referred to almost with affection during the recent war as 'Uncle Joe', and described by Roosevelt as 'a man I can do business with',[34] had lost his avuncular sheen.

By now Roosevelt had departed the scene and furthermore 'Uncle Joe' had stolen America's atomic secrets[35] and was tooled up with his own bomb. Business with Uncle Joe was turning out to be more difficult now that the mutual enemy, Hitler, had been disposed of. Indeed, there was mass hysteria about his ambitions. But cometh the hour cometh the man. Roosevelt might have been duped by Stalin at Yalta, but Senator Joseph McCarthy was made of sterner stuff.

Nobody exemplifies the *zeitgeist* better than McCarthy. Atypical of the Irish Catholic diaspora then, he adhered not to the Democratic but to the Republican Party and indeed to the right wing thereof. He was, furthermore, excessively demonstrative in milking his Catholicism and was the darling of their American Lordships.[36] McCarthy, the self-appointed scourge of all things 'un-American',[37] and a man who has done no credit to his Irish name, would keep America safe for God.

The underclasses of America would be spared the iniquity of 'socialised medicine'.

Ireland was perhaps the least likely place in the world to succumb to the charms of Moscow in 1950, but the price of freedom is eternal vigilance. John Charles McQuaid, Catholic Archbishop of Dublin, was nothing if not vigilant. While not exhibiting the florid paranoia of McCarthy, his mentality nevertheless was one of siege. Already entrenched for a decade and in a position of great power over the political apparatus, he was a stout defender of an obscurantist status quo. He was, of course, more temperate than McCarthy in his utterances, but one suspects that his thoughts, as indeed with the American Bishops, were not far removed. In 1951, in verbiage which is carefully crafted to appear reasonable, he admonishes the Taoiseach that any proposed health legislation should 'Respect in its principles and implementation the traditional life and spirit of our Christian people.'[38]

While these words, on their face value, seem benign and reasonable, their import was that the status quo was acceptable: that any importation of the liberal tendencies, then gaining traction elsewhere, would result in a ruinous descent into communism. As McCarthy would protect the American people from the Godless creed, so also would McQuaid not be found wanting in sparing 'our Christian people' from that menace.

THE SLEUTH OF FERNS

It is only normal to expect that a man who embarked on such a grandiose mission, espionage was after all the *leitmotif* of the time, would require his own intelligence gathering apparatus and so it came to pass. The Irish iteration of that scourge of communism, the dubious J. Edgar Hoover,[39] was to be none other than McQuaid's most trusted lieutenant, fellow traveller and kitchen cabinet colleague, the Bishop of Ferns, James Staunton. Staunton, on the instructions of McQuaid, set up and headed a committee[40] to monitor the activities of left wingers who might have dangerous notions about 'the traditional life and spirit' of the nation. Staunton did not need to resort to the electronic eavesdropping then in its infancy, but rather relied upon a fecundity of Catholics of conservative outlook whom he implanted in every suspect organisation.[41] Those spied upon were a pathetic rag tag and bobtail of the left and the exercise evokes more the farce of Graham Greene's *Our Man in Havana*[42] than of a le Carré thriller.

Not least among those attracting the attentions of what we might call Staunton's Committee on un-Irish activities was Noël Browne, Minister for Health.

SOCIAL ENGINEERING

A disadvantage for those, including the Minister for Health, who would wish to follow the British model of completely free healthcare was that England at this time was extremely dysfunctional. Having heroically won the war, it now seemed that the decaying empire was determined to lose the peace. It was easy, as the State increased its penetration into medicine, for conservative elements in Ireland to use the prevailing industrial chaos to damn, by association, the direction in which British society was going.

Nothing exemplified this road to hell better than the epochal cinematographic portrayal of the stereotypical anti-hero of the (slightly later) time, Mr Fred Kite in the movie *I'm Alright Jack*.[43] The tyrannical jumped up shop steward Kite (Peter Sellers), a metaphor for all denizens of the left, by his antics brought the whole industrial apparatus of the country to a stop. Although Kite was a fictional and comic character, the menace which he portrayed was real enough and continued for many years.

While Fred Kite was a caricature of the trade union attitude of the time, he reflected, more than a little, the attitude of the proletariat. This latter word enjoyed considerable currency in the regurgitations of the Moscowniks then, but one would search long to find a quotation where it tripped off the tongue of the Archbishop of Dublin, or his sleuth the Bishop of Ferns.

Exhausted by the war effort and the subsequent austerity, the English working man wanted to cash in his chips. He wanted a life of ease. He felt that the profits earned by the sweat of his brow should go towards his comfort and welfare rather than towards the perpetuation of an unproductive and effete elite which had long preyed upon him. He had a visceral rather than an intellectual appreciation of the struggle between capital and labour, between private and public. He was happy to leave the intellectual stuff to leftist elements of the intelligentsia and the press, who were better equipped to work out the details. He did however understand the role of anarchy in social engineering. A pragmatist rather than an ideologue, and not excessively preoccupied by social theory, he knew that he could stop the trains, put out the lights and close the mines – and his government knew this also. He could, at will, titrate into the social mix a whiff of revolution which had a most salutary effect upon the establishment.

In the prevailing atmosphere of cold war paranoia, with the memory of the slaughter of the Royal cousins by the Bolsheviks still fresh, the establishment decided, out of necessity rather than virtue, *sauve qui peut,* that it would have to give ground. This concession spawned a raft of 'progressive' measures not least among which was that *bête noir* of the Irish medical and ecclesiastical establishments, 'socialised medicine' – the free-for-all National Health Service.

These events, very close to home, were viewed with the greatest alarm by the Irish vested interests in medicine and the Church, who in matters of social policy much preferred the American approach of *laissez faire.* If Fred Kite had shown his face in America he would have been beaten off the streets by Pinkerton men.[44] Furthermore, in America unions and capital shared the same bed, often on terms of intimacy. In England they occupied opposite ends of the house and communicated by megaphone.

At the precise time under discussion, 1951, when hysteria about communism might reasonably have been considered already to have reached its zenith, it received a further boost. An espionage event of seismic proportions in England provided conservative elements in Ireland, ecclesiastical, medical and other, with ammunition to argue, and indeed with very little regret, that Perfidious Albion was finally on the road to perdition.

In May 1951 two renegades from the bosom of the British establishment, Guy Burgess and Donald Maclean, disappeared[45] and a few weeks later turned up in Moscow carrying a great bag of His Majesty's secrets. Britain, fearing that Burgess and McLean were merely the tip of the dissident iceberg, was in complete disarray. These defections to communism from the very heart of the British establishment, the *cause célèbre* of the time, must have afforded to right wing elements in Ireland – Church, State and medical – the greatest affirmation that they had been vindicated in circling the wagons against the iniquitous liberal contagion affecting the neighbouring island. Furthermore, they were now enabled to misrepresent what was in fact a diehard rearguard action against much needed medical reform, as motivated not by a desire to preserve their respective power, purse and positions, but rather as a bulwark against the menace of communism.

Those who controlled Ireland would see to it that Fred Kite, with all his works and pomps, including his free-for-all National Health Service, would remain confined to the other island.

3

NO BEVERIDGE, THANK YOU

So it was that Ireland at mid-twentieth century, with regard to planning a Health Service, was faced with a choice between State interventionism and *laissez faire*, a choice between active State intervention as advocated by Beveridge[46] in the UK and the American preference for *laissez faire* caricatured by the whacky John Birch Society[47] but enjoying much support in 'Middle America'. The Minister for Health, Noël Browne, embraced the former, and the medical establishment and the Catholic Church the latter.

The British National Health Service takes its origin from the highly interventionist Beveridge report of 1942. The report, with the exception of the British Medical Association, was received with acclaim. The attitude of the English Religious establishment is reflected by the Archbishop of Canterbury who, speaking of Beveridge, stated that it was 'the first time that anyone had set out to embody the whole spirit of the Christian ethic in an Act of Parliament'.[48]

This was in marked contrast to the attitude of the Catholic Archbishop of Dublin, John Charles McQuaid who, when the Minister for Health, Noël Browne, proposed an altogether more modest intervention, the Mother and Child Scheme in 1950, objected on the less than Christian and quite disingenuous grounds that, in order to implement it 'the State must levy a heavy tax on the whole community, by direct or indirect methods, independently of the necessity or desire of the citizens to use the facilities provided'.[49]

As already discussed, the British citizen, after the travails of war, was looking for a free lunch and it came in the form of a raft of 'progressive' measures which has come to be known as the Welfare State, the firstborn offspring of which was the National Health Service. The infant was welcomed into the world with great acclaim and its early growth and development were closely observed by all – not least those Herod-like[50] denizens of Church and medicine in Ireland who felt threatened by the new arrival. They conspired together that, in the event of the infant rearing his head in Ireland, it should be strangled at birth.

NO FREE LUNCH

The great problem with free lunches, however, is their price. And the price of the new Beveridge-inspired National Health Service soon emerged. There also emerged a new definition of the heretofore less than complicated word 'free'. The service would not, in fact, be free at all but would be – in a formula admirable for its creativity if not for its honesty – 'free at the point of delivery'. Remote from the point of delivery, however, the new service would be funded by pilfering weekly, by law, every wage packet in the land with a special health levy. To his credit the Archbishop of Dublin, with his 'heavy tax on the whole community', was prepared to call a spade a spade while the British Government was regaling its population with nuance and sleight of hand.

According to the credo of conservative American non-interventionists, often of a religious bent, the market, if left to itself, will deal effectively with almost every problem of society and any occasional area in which it is found wanting will be sorted out by God. Any unfortunates who fall off the wagon of prosperity have only themselves to blame, and any intervention by the State towards their support will serve only further to encourage their delinquency. Yet again the strictures of St Luke regarding our old friend Lazarus are cast aside by these American exponents of conservative Christian non-interventionism. These ardent followers of Jesus proceed in *a la carte* mode and think little of the Biblical advice, 'If you have two coats give one to the poor.'[51]

Masters of doublethink, these plutocrats have forty coats, pray with piety, thump the Bible and never yield a stitch.

HIPPOCRATES IN AMERICA

The American doctor and his professional organisations at mid-twentieth century considered the socialisation of medicine to be an anathema and entirely inconsistent with American values – a violation of the much trumpeted 'American Way'. He – for it was then most often a male – enjoyed a position of considerable privilege and comfort in society and felt his interests were best served by preservation of the status quo, that is, private medicine. True, like doctors elsewhere, he had taken the Hippocratic Oath and certainly the concepts contained therein governed him in areas relating to matters of decorum. Such decorum, much taught in medical schools, underpinned the gravitas with which the medical profession would wish to be perceived. Hippocrates, however, although he antedated Jesus Christ by several centuries,[52] is no less vulnerable to mischievous selective citation and some of his ideas regarding the interface between medicine and economics did not entirely chime with 'the American Way'. For decorum Hippocrates was your man, but what did he know of business? And as we have seen, American medicine was, after all, a business. A business sells its product for the best price it can get; it does not give it away. Not to put too fine a point on it, the American doctor felt that his material prosperity, and indeed his independence, were likely to be in inverse proportion to the level of government involvement in medicine.

In Ireland events would show that the medical establishment viewed this inverse relationship with an equally jaundiced eye.

Beveridge is, politically, the polar opposite of *laissez faire*. The respective ideologies are those of Robin Hood and Scrooge. Beveridge was a great liberal economic thinker of the interbellum years while the essence of the American thinking was that of the Cold War warrior. Beveridge was offering a policy of maximum state intervention in healthcare. While not wishing in any way to categorise him as a plagiarist, one is tempted to observe that his ideas bore more than a passing resemblance to those articulated 2,000 years before by one Jesus Christ – a point which was not lost on the Archbishop of Canterbury but found little resonance with the Archbishop of Dublin.

Here, then, we have a very secular England, notwithstanding the enigma of its established Church, proposing a plan for the health of its people which might have been devised by Jesus Christ Himself – but making no mention of the man from Nazareth. Meanwhile, in the land of the free and Joe McCarthy, the Messiah is widely trumpeted. There is much Halleluiah. America takes its opium but not its social or healthcare policy from 'the Good Book'.

But what of little mid-Atlantic Ireland in all of this? She was still struggling to shake off post-imperial torpor and poverty, with her commerce controlled by her erstwhile rulers, the nation of shopkeepers.[53] Would she opt for Beveridge or a less interventive formula, or would she perhaps fudge the issue? Would the Irish political leadership have the independence of mind and the vision to think its way through this medico-socio-economic and ideological maze in order to provide for its people an indigenously conceived, culturally suitable and affordable and equitable system of healthcare? Most important of all, would the body politic seek disinterested advice, or would it lend its ear to the tendentious utterings of vested interest?

The answer to this latter question forms the substance to the remainder of this book: it is not an edifying tale.

4

'THE CANCER OF SOCIALISED MEDICINE'

There is little doubt as to where the Irish Medical Association (IMA) stood in the ideological debate. Happily, for the historical record, the position of the IMA is encapsulated precisely in a memorandum (1951) to Government setting out its opinion and suggestions for the future of the Irish Health Service. A copy of this memorandum, like much else of the time, found its way into the admirable Dublin Diocesan Archive.[54] While there is much in the document that is rational, its main thrust is a blueprint for the material prosperity of the medical profession. On the hot topic of the State involvement in medicine it lapses into hysteria.

The section headed 'Dangers to be guarded against' is worthy of quotation in full, and of some analysis. These 'dangers' are very many indeed, leaving the reader wondering as to who indeed was endangered.

THE DANGERS

> Wholesale and immediate National Health Service on a compulsory contributory basis, i.e. similar to the British Scheme. However this be brought about the overall cost would be enormous. The various objections, ethical, financial and moral have been re-iterated by leading sociologists, medical and political leaders.

> Gradual extension of state control to all medical services. This Fabian technique has been employed in this country for many years and resulted in the recent crisis in health affairs. It takes the form of extending the genuine need of public health preventative services to the domain of curative services; of starvation of voluntary services and boosting of State services; of control of more and more of the profession by whole-time appointments and salaries; of State advertising of State services and denigration of the voluntary services; and finally of a conditioning of the people to accept the 'paternalism' of the State in all medical matters.

> This form of State control is more insidious, and in the long run it is also more expensive. Owing to the fact that the cost is met from central and local taxation rather than from a personal contribution it is politically more popular. It is to be noted that it has led in this country to a far greater control of certain medical services by lay bureaucrats than the more radical system in Britain. An extension of the system would lead to huge administrative costs and lay control of medical services.

The medical leadership wanted to keep the State out of medicine at all costs and the tendentious arguments advanced above are clear enough, if for the most part disingenuous. The 'Fabian technique' by which the society[55] of that name had, by a gradualist and thoroughly democratic approach, advanced State involvement in Britain, is disparaged as a threat to 'ethical' and 'moral' values. This reference shows how attuned the medical leadership was to political events in Britain.

The State, according to this analysis by the Irish medical establishment, should confine itself to 'public health and preventative services' but should back off any involvement in the practice of clinical medicine. It is an extraordinary assertion, not comfortable for a medical writer to read today, that the State in a parliamentary democracy should not have any involvement in 'curative services' and that the 'boosting of State services' should be represented as iniquitous and a blow against 'ethical' and 'moral' norms. It should be remembered that almost all 'voluntary services' (which could be read as Voluntary Hospitals) were either owned directly by the Church or vicariously controlled by it. It was clear that in any standoff between Church and State in the area of medicine, the doctors would be on the side of the angels. The medical establishment had little difficulty in sowing alarm in the minds of Their Lordships by convincing them that the flagship hospitals which they controlled were, as a consequence of this 'Fabian' conspiracy, about to suffer 'starvation'.

The essence of the IMA argument, and that of its Episcopal co-conspirators, was that clinical independence would not survive the proposed introduction of 'whole time appointments and salaries'. This decidedly unflattering opinion of the profession is deserving of some examination.

In contemporary America, with the introduction of 'Obamacare', the right wing is again screaming foul. It should be noted, however, that in that country many of the finest medical institutions, which score most highly in annual 'league tables'[56] of performance published by the press, have for many years employed their internationally renowned senior doctors on the basis of what the IMA disparaged as 'whole time appointments and salaries'. These doctors are not robbed of their clinical independence by their employer and it is for the most part they, rather than those who work privately and independently, who lead scientific advances and progress for patients.

The virulent antipathy of senior doctors towards any organisation of medical services involving 'whole-time appointments and salaries' is emblematic of the time. It is clear that the IMA regarded the concept of professionalism as incompatible with working for an employer, even one providing medical services and being paid a salary. This must surely have been offensive to the many other salaried professionals in Ireland who were working hard to build up the still nascent State. In particular it would do little for the digestion of highly professional civil servants in the Department of Health, who were in frequent contact with the organisation which used such condescending language and disparaged them as 'lay bureaucrats'.

In passing it is relevant to mention that Irish medical schools of the time (c. 1950) were badly neglected. Certain senior clinical staff in these schools were to the fore in resisting State intervention and doubtless as role models inculcated this attitude in their juniors. They were, it would seem, more exercised by their efforts to frustrate the laudable plans of the Minister for Health than in looking to the preservation and standards of their own medical schools. This neglect had brought the schools disgrace and close to perdition. They were staffed mainly by part time poorly remunerated clinical appointees, dependent for their living on practice (mainly private) in several locations. This had led to a marked deterioration in academic standards and structures, drawing censure from international licensing bodies.[57] American inspecting bodies were particularly censorious and recognition was withdrawn. The ignominious situation had been allowed to develop such that Irish doctors' degrees were not recognised abroad. This mandated emergency salvage action, prescribed neither by the doyens of medicine nor the universities but, to the shame of both, by outsiders. This, demanded by outsiders, was precisely the form of action that the IMA and their Church backers had resisted on 'ethical' and 'moral' grounds – 'whole-time appointments and salaries'.

The IMA memorandum goes on to cite no less an authority than *The Economist*, which was allowing itself to lapse into the convenient belief that the British free-for-all National Health Service would collapse in ruins under the financial pressure.

The Economist of 11 March 1950 said:

The only way in which the Scheme [i.e. National Health Service] can be saved is to abandon altogether the principle that it should be entirely free. Exactly how a charge should be imposed will need to be carefully thought out (there would certainly have to be a means test to avoid hardship). But it has become quite obvious to all but the most prejudiced that a charge is the only way to bring home financial realities to patients and practitioners as well as to restore the health of the service itself.

The IMA memorandum reaches a crescendo of hysteria with a dire warning, worthy of Jeremiah[58] himself, regarding 'the dangers of bureaucracy and the cancer of socialised medicine'.

The comparison of publicly provided medical services to the most dreaded disease of cancer is beyond reprehensible, represents the worst kind of scaremongering and is entirely unworthy of the Hippocratic profession.

The IMA prophesy of doom ends with the admonition 'that the individual should be encouraged to escape by his own efforts from the toils of regimentation in medical treatment'. This latter sentiment is spectacularly lacking in vision. The great effectiveness of modern medicine is largely attributable to the structure and predictability provided by training programmes, algorithms, protocols and standardised procedures. While these diagnostic and treatment pathways are not without tedium, and indeed do on occasion amount to regimentation, the expectation that such 'toils' could be avoided in a modern and complex world was at best naïve and at worst disingenuous.

5

Two Strong Men Stand
Face to Face

In order to understand the impending drama it is necessary to
reflect somewhat on the two great antagonists involved and
what made them each as they were – John Charles McQuaid
and Noël C. Browne.

Celtic Talleyrand

McQuaid was the ultimate Catholic chauvinist. He was from an
obscure place made famous by Percy French, Cootehill, County
Cavan, where his father was a general practitioner. Because of
his formidable organisational talents, his rise in the Church had
been meteoric. He was consecrated Archbishop of Dublin, the
most powerful ecclesiastical office in the land, in 1940 at the age
of a vigorous 45 years. His reign, for such it is appropriate to
call it, was to last for 32 years. He would prove to be the nearest
thing to a Celtic Talleyrand[59] that Ireland has produced.

In general intellectuality was regarded with suspicion by the
Irish Catholic elite of 1950. Academic learning, while it has of
course immense value for civilisation, was preferred to original
thought. And well might the Church of that time be pleased
with this formula. Globalisation was after all not invented by
Coca Cola, Toyota or Morgan Sachs Bank but by the Church
of Rome which rejoiced in styling itself as 'universal'. Original
thinking, however, can be troublesome and its exponents are

employed sparingly by global organisations, and only at the very top. Better to rely on people slightly below this level who are generally characterised as clever – high academic achievers but spared the burden of too much original thought.

The received wisdom of the Catholic Church had been refined over two millennia and had been successful without parallel. During that time empires of this world came and went in ever diminishing cycles, but the Rock of Peter stood firm. The leadership in Rome kept an iron grip on the organisation in the manner of an American big city political machine like Tammany Hall[60] or the Prendergasts[61] in Kansas City – both Irish Catholic diaspora manifestations. The objective was institutional preservation. McQuaid was the ideal man to implement this policy.

The approach of the Church, although global, was entirely different from that of global businesses. The latter know that change will come at them and they must adapt to it or disappear. They must take risks; risk is safer than no risk. For the Church, and John Charles McQuaid, values were absolute. Their view was, perhaps understandably, that our product has endured for 2,000 years – nineteen centuries more than Coca Cola.

This approach is hard to rebut when things are going well and in 1950 the Catholic Church generally, and in Ireland in particular, was rampant. The institution worked and the evidence was everywhere to be seen. The Archbishop of Dublin, therefore, in his obdurate resistance to social change, could offer – indeed before its time using the dreary correctspeak of modern medical theorists – that his position was 'evidence-based'. And the message from Rome was, you are doing fine, maintain course, no change please.

John Charles McQuaid valued the approbation of Rome above all else. This ultramontanist outlook caused him predominantly to respond to stimuli from Rome with less regard for local opinion. It was widely accepted in Ireland that he aspired to the red hat. He was determined in all that he did to demonstrate to the Vatican mandarins that he was made of the right stuff for this elevation – the consummation of all his ambitions. He believed that by the exemplary destruction of the Minister for Health, and that by keeping the State out of medicine, he would further endear himself to the Vatican insiders.

Nobody exemplifies the smouldering historic resentment of the disproportionate power and position of the minority Protestant community in Ireland better than Archbishop McQuaid. His mission was to redress that imbalance. His methods would not be delicate.

The enigmatically named Church of Ireland was anything but that. From its minority position it had long held sway in business, commerce, the professions, the prestige of its church buildings and much else. The Church of (the majority of) the people of Ireland played second fiddle. This anomaly was now, through the democratic process, incrementally correcting itself. It is in the nature of such corrections that there are often elements of over-swing. The Archbishop of Dublin was a manifestation of this phenomenon, a metaphor for the intolerances which bespattered the Catholic liturgy.[62] A man of more vision than John Charles McQuaid might have realised that magnanimity rather than triumphalism would have been a better path to a happy equilibrium.

But the Archbishop had been forged in the sectarian furnace of the Ulster border country where magnanimity in his youth would have been scarce enough. Intolerance seems to have been seared into his soul. He would have little affection for planters, covenanters, hyphenated types and suchlike, and when his intellect secured for him a position of power, he would give them little quarter. He wasted his God-given intellectual gifts and practiced more the philosophy of Shylock – 'I will feed fat the ancient grudge I bear him'[63] – than that of the founder of Christianity. Still smarting on one cheek he was not a man, as his divine mentor had suggested, to turn the other. A well-educated man, he felt mistakenly that the tide of history was running his way and he would ride the wave. Being an ardent admirer of Seneca,[64] he felt that the asceticism and restraint advocated by that noble Roman would be a suitable prescription to moderate the tendency to excess of the Irish people. He was scarcely wrong in this, but ironically, such an analysis might more expectedly have come from a Protestant Bishop.

One of McQuaid's earliest thrusts was at Trinity College (University of Dublin). This great institution, with its portals guarded by Burke and Goldsmith, while ancient and venerable was, alas, essentially Protestant. It was the Archbishop's *bête noire*. McQuaid vigorously enforced the ban on Catholics attending there.[65] This academy was alright for the licentious antics of J. P. Dunleavy and his 'Ginger Man',[66] but no place for young Catholics and most particularly not for young Catholic doctors in the making. Medical ethics, as taught in such a place of Reformation and iniquity, would not have the same predictability as in institutions where the agents of Drumcondra ruled.

Two Cathedrals and a Church

The Archbishop of Dublin, a Counter-Reformation man if ever there was one, notwithstanding the asceticism which he would prescribe for the Irish nation, was a great admirer of the extravagant exuberance of Renaissance Italian churches. It must, therefore, have galled him more than a little to behold his nemeses, Their Protestant Lordships, ensconced in the finest cathedrals and churches in Dublin, and indeed elsewhere throughout the country. He, meanwhile, had to plant his chair in the somewhat enigmatically named Pro-Cathedral.

There was, of course, a roof over the Archbishop's head in the Pro-Cathedral but it was scarcely a place of pilgrimage. Meanwhile, the tourists and literary cognoscenti from afar came to pay homage to the shrine of Dean Swift at St Patrick's Cathedral. Busloads of left-footed Americans were uncomprehending that St Patrick's Cathedral, unlike its namesake in New York, was not a Catholic place. There were no bus tours of literary groupies or cognoscenti to His Grace's place, hemmed into the tight confines of Marlborough Street.

And worse again the minority religion possessed, on the Archbishop's doorstep, not one High Kirk but two.

On their way to St Patrick's Cathedral, travellers would happen upon the glorious Christchurch Cathedral and learn, *mirabile dictu*, that this also was a Protestant place. Two magnificent medieval cathedrals, within spitting distance of each other, serving a platoon of Protestants while the massed divisions of Catholics, and their fearless general in Drumcondra, had to make do with the merely neo-classical non-cathedral in Marlborough Street.

There was one last piece of outlandishness which must have irked the Archbishop and totally confounded the visitors. They would be told that St Laurence O'Toole, a Pre-Reformation (Catholic) prelate, had built Christchurch which, along with much else, was confiscated during the Reformation but was still claimed by the Catholic Archdioceses of Dublin as the seat of the Archbishop. The Catholic Archdioceses, meanwhile, pending restitution of its legitimate seat, installed Laurence as the patron of the Pro-Cathedral in Marlborough Street – notwithstanding that he was equally revered by the Protestants. Symbolically, the Catholic Archdioceses would stay in Marlborough Street – in its Pro-Cathedral rather than a full cathedral – until it could reclaim the heritage of St Laurence O'Toole. His Grace John Charles McQuaid, Archbishop of Dublin, would have to tough it out in his Pro-Cathedral – waiting for Godot.

Nor was the architectural deprivation of the majority Catholic community confined to the nation's capital. Travelling in rural Ireland, and particularly in delightful coastal villages in the south west, one comes upon a strange phenomenon. Adorning the village, in prime position, is a beautiful ancient stone-built church. Sporting its credentials and its schedule of services on its neat notice board, it is immediately recognisable as 'Church of Ireland'. Scarcely troubled by 'a platoon' its gravel path is not well trodden. But where is the Church of the vast majority of the people of Ireland? Often it is found in desolate places, sticking up incongruously and isolated from its patrons a mile or two outside the village – a mile which, at the time of building, the worshipers would have had to trudge in all weathers. Architecturally undistinguished and rarely adorned by tower or steeple, such sequestrated churches were emblematic of 'the ancient grudge' to which the Archbishop of Dublin was prisoner – a grudge which was now damaging the country and the development of its Health Service.

None of this is offered as an excuse for the behaviour and attitudes of the Archbishop of Dublin, but it does afford some insight into the genesis of such attitudes. His personality, experience and conditioning did not allow him to overcome 'the ancient grudge'. Unable to find magnanimity when he got the upper hand he lapsed into triumphalism. He was no Nelson Mandela, or perhaps more to the point, he was no Gordon Wilson.[67]

Good Luck, Bad Luck

Noël Browne grew up in the west of Ireland in difficult economic circumstances. In his early years he was a product of Irish National and Christian Brothers schools and his personality and politics were determined by the hardships of his family at this time. Such a family could not aspire to the world of Clongowes Wood or Blackrock College, both enjoyed by his nemesis McQuaid. The death of his father from tuberculosis resulted in his removal to relatives in England, a blessing in disguise – although well disguised at the time.

In England, by his academic brilliance, he gained scholarship entry into a Jesuit fee paying 'public school'[68] where he excelled. Thereafter, as a result of philanthropy, he was enabled to study medicine at Trinity College Dublin whence he graduated in 1942. After postgraduate work in England he returned to Ireland and entered politics. He became Minister for Health in the first inter-party government in 1948. His agenda was to redress those miseries which had plagued his childhood – the national scourges of tuberculosis and poverty.

Noël Browne's rise was no less meteoric than that of his great adversary, McQuaid. Even before the controversy, however, he was by personality a somewhat remote and isolated figure. This was exemplified by his penchant, during the composition of official cabinet and other photographs, of placing himself on the periphery of the group and more often than not – and perhaps not by chance – on the left. He displayed some of the vulnerability of the straggler.

Of significance is that in his correspondence at this time the Minister wrote his departmental address and the date in Irish, something which neither the Taoiseach nor the Archbishop were doing. In doing so he was making a clear statement for the benefit of his parliamentary colleagues and the many others of jingoistic nationalist tendency who did not love him. He was obviously sensitive of his provenance in this regard since both his father and grandfather had been members of the Royal Irish Constabulary. It does him little credit that he fails to mention this in his autobiography. The belated memoir might be allowed understandable lapses of memory, but one does not forget one's father's occupation. He felt defensively obliged on many occasions to reassert his Irishness. He was in effect saying, I am as Irish and as patriotic, and indeed perhaps more so, than the rest of you. Indeed, he had often been accused, by innuendo or overtly, of being otherwise. His detractors in this regard exhibited the prejudice which the ignorant sometimes visit upon those who are different, and particularly on those whom they perceive to be different and superior. In this regard Noël Browne was damned on both counts.

To the Irish perception, nothing makes a man different more than the way he speaks – his accent. Returning from his English diaspora where he had spent his formative educational years, Noël Browne spoke, as do many such Irish, with a conspicuously different hybrid accent. But this accent differed from that of most other returning Irish: it was not working class. His English public school, albeit a minor one and Catholic, had conditioned him to speak beautifully but not without a hint of condescension and superiority. This self-assured aura, while falling well short of the superciliousness of Eton or Harrow, or for that matter of Stoneyhurst or Ampleforth, was sufficient to raise the dander of certain bumpkin elements who inhabited the benches in Leinster House in 1950. Such elements were easy prey to be turned against the Minister by powerful prelates or doyen doctors.

The Minister for Health was sensitive to his incompetence in Irish, the official language of the State. In this regard he was little different from many of his tormentors but he did a remarkable thing. He took himself off to an Irish speaking area in the remote west of the country, where he spent time among the ordinary people and learned their vernacular. Thus becoming competent in the language, he surpassed many who made their living from it, and left his bumpkin detractors for dead.

Rather as having had a good war has made the reputation of many a politician, the war on tuberculosis made the reputation of Noël Browne. There was, however, more than a little luck in this. It should be remembered that antituberculous drugs arrived at a most opportune time for him. Streptomycin had been discovered in 1943[69] and had worked its way into clinical practice in Ireland during Browne's tenure in the Department of

Health. He made the drug available to all free of charge but any Minister would probably have done this. While streptomycin was epoch-making in its effect, it was the structure and organisation brought to its application by Noël Browne that made his programme a resounding success. The Department of Health, in the almost seven decades that have intervened, has not seen another Minister possessed of this focus and vision.

Up until the time he jousted with the Archbishop of Dublin, Noël Browne, after a difficult start, had become extremely lucky in life. He had been plucked from relative poverty and privately and expensively educated in England. His excellent God-given brain made him an avid recipient for this learning. Philanthropy had put him through medical school – albeit one in which Their Lordships the Bishops had no confidence and which was detested by Archbishop McQuaid. He overcame tuberculous disease personally, against the odds. He was appointed as the *enfant terrible* of the cabinet at an impossibly young age. He was given the portfolio which he craved. And then, right on cue, streptomycin arrived. Up until now every time he threw a dice it came up six. It could not last.

Unfortunately, the Minister's Mother and Child Scheme did not meet with the approval of the all powerful Catholic establishment. He was now dicing with the Archbishop of Dublin – an unwise diversion in 1950 – and his run of sixes has come to an end.

6

A LETTER FROM FERNS

While the position of the Irish Medical Association on the State's proposed penetration of medicine was one of unequivocal opposition, the Catholic Hierarchy's attitude was transmitted to the Government with even more implacable clarity.

The Secretary to the Hierarchy at that time was the Bishop of a dioceses then obscure but now better known – Ferns. Their Lordships were in the habit, when they foregathered, of referring on occasion to each other informally by their diocesan moniker. It therefore fell to 'Ferns', in the person of Bishop James Staunton, to communicate to Government the collective views of the Hierarchy on various matters – to give the politicians their riding orders, so to speak. Not least among the matters exercising the Hierarchy at this time was the proposed Mother and Child Scheme and its promoter the Minister for Health.

It is significant that 'Ferns' did not write to the Minister for Health. That would have been *infra dignitatem*. The Hierarchy were, after all, the head of the Church, the real government.

Staunton was instructed to write to the Taoiseach.

This was no ordinary missive. The Archbishop of Dublin, a man unaccustomed to such trivial tasks, acted as courier: he handed the letter to the Taoiseach. The signal was clear. The Bishops were roused.

The envelope containing the Ferns letter from the Hierarchy which was handed by McQuaid to the Taoiseach has a resonance in modern Ireland. It was, of course, less grimy in content than the many that were passed to politicians by the lobbyists and spivs of the Celtic Tiger era. Nor was the Taoiseach, who was an honourable man, one to be bought by hard currency. The Archbishop, furthermore, would be aghast at the suggestion that he was doing anything wrong. But therein lies the rub. Both men thought that their actions were proper – honourable men both.

But the envelope was passed with the clear objective of furtively influencing the decisions of government. The currency contained in the envelope was not of the hard vulgar monetary kind, but it was equally persuasive and in the event altogether more effective.

Nothing captures the zeitgeist of 1950 in Ireland like that letter (Appendix 1). Readers in the twenty-first century, if they are young or indeed middle aged, and who cannot or do not wish to believe that it was as described here, should read the letter. It is likely that some medical people of sincere Catholic faith will disagree with the analysis presented here; they also should read the letter. Most of the clergy of that day have been swept away by time. It is unlikely that their successors have been objectively educated in these uncomfortable matters in the seminary; if they are sceptical they also should read the letter.

It is October 1950. The negotiations between the Department of Health and the IMA on the introduction of a no means test free-for-all Mother and Child Scheme have reached an acrimonious impasse. The medical establishment has run a vigorous campaign but has not yet overcome Minister Browne and blocked his scheme. Nevertheless, the campaign now promises to be a resounding success because the Bishops are in the fray. Their Lordships are representing the issue as one of 'faith and morals', in addition to insisting that the scheme is acceptable to them only if it is not free-for-all: it must be means tested. What began life as a well-meaning and much-needed measure to improve the health and safety of pregnant women and their babies has, contrary to all reasonable expectation, morphed into a monstrous attack on the moral fibre of the nation.

The medical establishment could now relax. The running would henceforth be made by their Lordships and their main man in Drumcondra. The doyens of medicine would, vicariously through the Bishops, grossly pervert the legitimate business of the State to the detriment of its citizens – their patients.

And so to the letter from Ferns of 10 October 1950:

> The Archbishops and Bishops of Ireland, at their meeting on October 10th, had under consideration the proposals for Mother and Child health service and other kindred health services.

The Bishops met on 10 October and the letter was shot off immediately on the same day. Many a wiser head might have decided to sleep on it. The Catholic Hierarchy of 1950, however, saw little need for such circumspection.

Use of the word 'kindred' here is most interesting. The Minister had made it clear in all his utterances and documentation that the proposed Mother and Child Service would be clearly circumscribed: it was designed to deal with a specific and scandalous problem. The word 'kindred', however, implies such things as family, progeny etc. It was being made clear that the Bishops anticipated that there would be a spawn of further related, and to them equally undesirable, measures, increasing the State's penetration into what they considered to be their own domain. The implication is clear: prevention is better than cure – they would stop the rot now, nip it in the bud.

> They recognise that the proposals are motivated by a sincere desire to improve the public health, but they feel

> bound by their office to consider whether the proposals
> are in accordance with Catholic moral teaching.

This is faint praise indeed and addressed to the head of Government is patronising in the extreme. It is, however, as close to approbation as the letter gets: from here on it is all downhill.

'Catholic moral teaching' should, of course, without question, be the business of Catholic Bishops. The law of the land, however, was an entirely different question and this Jeffersonian[70] principle they repeatedly did not or would not grasp. Indeed, it is likely that they did not believe in the separation of Church and State. To control the Church was good indeed: to control the Church which controlled the State was altogether better.

> ... the powers taken by the State in the proposed Mother
> and Child Health Service are in direct opposition to the
> rights of the family and the individual.

The Catholic Hierarchy have always been commendable in their defence of the family. They continue, in the modern era, to stand their traditional ground on various improvised redefinitions of that word. This is how they should function. They should, however, confine their persuasions to their own followers and not, as undoubtedly they did in 1950, and on more than a few occasions since, try to bully the State. Indeed, the suggestion that the proposed improved Health Service would damage 'the rights of the family' and the individual was an extraordinary conclusion and now makes the Bishops look silly. This was a deception by the Bishops of their followers and a betrayal of their trust. It is clear that the service would do exactly the opposite. It is clear also that the Hierarchy, in striving to prevent this benevolent measure, were straying far from the path of Jesus Christ, and the doctors in abetting them from that of Hippocrates. Indeed, it is tempting to offer that it would have caused the former, if He had not risen from it on the third day, to turn in His grave.

The language then becomes less temperate as 'Ferns' ramps up his onslaught.

> If adopted in law they would constitute a ready-made instrument for future totalitarian aggression.

He has somewhat lost the run of himself. His verbiage is typical of the time. He is using the language of war – the hot one recently finished, and the cold one, against dreaded communism, now raging.

The Hierarchy were declaring war against the Government.

It is difficult, such was the almost trivial nature of the *casus belli*, not to suspect that their Lordships wanted to pick a fight. They had since independence been dealing with compliant conservative Governments. This coalition Government, however, contained suspect feisty leftish elements, not least of whom was the Minister for Health. The Minister's Mother and Child Service proposal, and his obdurate adherence to it contrary to Episcopal 'advice', was an early indication that, if this measure were enacted, the writ of the Hierarchy might not run as smoothly as before. It is difficult to escape the conclusion that it was this fear, rather than any concern for mothers and children, that got their Lordships and their main man in Drumcondra so exercised. They decided that they would attack the Minister in order to prevent 'totalitarian aggression' and in so doing employed that very tactic. It would be total war, a fight to the finish.

> The right to provide for the health of children belongs to parents, not to the State. The State should supplement not supplant.

On the face of it this passage seems reasonable enough. Is His Lordship of Ferns however not perhaps using the word 'right' where the word 'duty' might be more appropriate? To suggest that parents were to be deprived of any right whatsoever was a nonsensical red herring, and unworthy. The State was, rather, proposing to provide the means to help parents towards the better discharge of their duties to their children. Indeed, to 'supplement' rather than 'supplant' was precisely what the State was proposing. The truth, however, was getting lost in the fog of verbal warfare. A service which by any yardstick should be seen as increasing citizens' rights was disingenuously represented, to Their Lordships' credulous followers, as diminishing them.

Ireland was poor in 1950 and many of its citizens were dirt poor. While poverty is, of course, relative to context and not easy to define, misery was everywhere to be seen. Although the Church concerned itself more with the spiritual than the economic, the Bishop of Ferns in his letter to the Taoiseach ventured to quantify what the Hierarchy considered to be the extent of this poverty.

> It [the state] may help indigent or neglectful parents; it may not deprive 90 per cent of parents of their rights because of 10 per cent of neglectful or necessitous parents.

Here then we have it in the starkest possible terms. The Hierarchy are, in menacing terms, telling the Government what it 'may' and 'may not' do. It has gauged that the Government, for electoral reasons, will not have the nerve to stand up to Their Lordships.

Extraordinary also was the figure of 10 per cent for poverty. Even when compared to war-ravaged Europe this figure was a gross and cynical underestimate, particularly for urban areas. The 'Echo Boy' in Cork was barefoot in winter.[71] He was the visible (and audible) tip of an iceberg of deprivation. He was of course at the Lazarus end of the economic spectrum – more the preoccupation, it would seem, of the Minister than the Bishops. Notwithstanding that it is taught as a subject in seminaries, the logic of why putting shoes on the 10 per cent would threaten the rights of the 90 per cent is not made clear. Indeed, there is more than a hint that the Hierarchy considered the miseries of children to be due in equal measure to 'neglectful' and 'necessitous' parents – a pedantic distinction which would be lost on the 'Echo Boy'.

This was excellent right wing stuff, the antithesis of Beveridge. Sooner or later, however, the mundane matter of money would have to be broached: this, after all, was the main concern of the doyens of medicine who had forged the Episco-Medical alliance.

> It is not sound social policy to impose a State medical service on the whole community on the pretext of relieving the necessitous 10 per cent from the so called indignity of a means test.

In economic, social and philosophical terms there is much sense in this statement – taken at its face value. The means test, an intrusive inquiry into how much money a person has, has always been looked upon in Ireland by trade unions and the left generally with the same affection which has been reserved for Oliver Cromwell, Charles Trevelyan and the Black and Tans. This is hypocrisy. The people have always shown themselves to be capable of swallowing 'the so called indignity' when there is something to be got gratis. Trade union opposition to means testing is ideological – a matter of dogma. Hypocrisy concerning means testing transcends all social barriers – the populist but expensive measure of issuing medical cards to all septuagenarians bears this out. When the benefit was withdrawn in the year 2009 because of financial meltdown, the well-heeled, indeed millionaires, joined the more deserving and took to the streets (indeed on the 'free travel') to protest the loss of their rights. The rights which the Bishops, implausibly, in 1950 said would be denied by the provision of a universal measure were, the citizens decided, equally denied by the withdrawal of a similar measure half a century later. Indeed, to convince oneself that the rights of the individual could be violated by providing a much needed benefit to her, required a measure of doublethink beyond the ordinary citizen. But the Bishops knew best.

The verb 'impose' is chosen with some mischief. The intention of the Minister for Health was to provide not to impose. The Irish people, rendered truculent by close to a millennium of foreign domination, were calculated not to take kindly to the notion of imposition. Such things as taxes, penalties and sentences were imposed. The Bishops were in fact saying that the Minister's scheme was an imposition – and the people trusted their Bishops.

It is extraordinary that the Hierarchy allowed themselves to become so hung up on the means test. It is, after all, a simple measure of how much money one has: it has no moral dimension. Perish the thought, however, that their Lordships should be seen to concern themselves with crude matters related to money. The issue must be dressed up as a moral one. The sheep must be given wolf's clothing.

> The right to provide for the physical education of children belongs to the family and not to the State. Experience has shown that physical or health education is closely interwoven with important moral questions on which the Catholic Church has definite teaching.

Again there is the word 'right' used disingenuously to suggest undermining of the family. Again, also, Their Lordships seek to define and limit the role of the State. What they believe in is a weak State, a strong Church – theocracy. One can almost hear the echo from Drumcondra: *L'État, cèst moi.*[72]

'Health education' in Ireland in 1950 was in a deplorable state. Families were in dire need of input from the State but the Bishops portrayed the Minister's proposal as an intrusion. In reality, it was altogether less of an intrusion than when an ambulance arrived at the family home to remove, by consent or compulsion, for sequestration in a sanatorium, a case of open tuberculosis – a common event.

The Church, of course, had no 'definite teaching' on tuberculosis: it could after all only kill the body. But could childbearing not also kill the body if not properly attended? Should the State not equally intervene to improve the chances of mother and child? According to the Bishop of Ferns, absolutely not. It would appear that there were 'important moral questions' related specifically to the matter of mothers and babies which rendered their pathologies and maladies apart from all other. The logic appeared to run that, certainly with tuberculosis, and indeed with childbearing, you could lose your body. You could, however, with the latter, if you ignored certain 'moral questions', compound the catastrophe by also losing your immortal soul. 'Ferns', his argument lacking substance, was falling back on good old fire and brimstone.

> Education in regard to motherhood includes instruction in regard to sex relations, chastity and marriage. The State has no competence to give instruction in such matters. We regard with the greatest apprehension the proposal to give local medical officers the right to tell Catholic girls and women how they should behave in regard to this sphere of conduct at once so delicate and sacred.

The 'local medical officer', although he or she was and to a large degree remains fundamental to clinical medicine in Ireland, is diminished by this paragraph. He is referred to not as a doctor but as a 'medical officer' – a mere functionary of the State. There is more than a suggestion that the fellow is not to be trusted, particularly with regard to 'important moral questions'. These doctors, however, were regarded in the highest possible esteem by their local communities and gave dedicated service, often for small reward; indeed, payment in kind was commonplace.

Doctors were generally perceived as doing no more than applying advances in scientific knowledge to the benefit of patients. Doctors, then as now, considered it their role to advise, to provide information, to furnish an opinion. The introduction of the Minister's scheme would not have changed this advisory role but would rather have enabled doctors to implement it to better effect. The doctor, after all, is a repository of biological knowledge and the 'such matters', which so exercised their Lordships, were biological. Why should the doctor's discharge of that for which he had been trained cause the Bishops 'the greatest apprehension'. Only those in fact who were themselves accustomed to telling 'Catholic girls and women how they should behave' could have expected doctors to do likewise.

A significant factor in the Bishops' reaction was the Church's instinctive distrust of science. The world was entering a period of accelerated scientific advancement. Although many thinkers see little conflict between scientific insight and religious belief, the Bishops were less sanguine: they had always relied heavily on mystery rather than reason. The demystifying effect of scientific discovery had the potential to deprive them of many of the levers with which they had controlled society. While scientific advances in medicine were seen as God-sent by the people, conservative Church elements were less reassured and viewed such developments, particularly in the area of reproduction, with suspicion and on occasions with hostility. They saw such progress as erosive of their control.

And there was worse. The Minister for Health, a scientifically trained doctor, and a suspect one to boot, was proposing to combine science with increased State intervention. Their Lordships would have worked out that, in many democratic societies, the powers of religion and State exist in inverse proportion. There was only so much power to go around and up until now they had enjoyed a disproportionate share. The unhappy concordance of scientific debunking and a muscular State filled them with consternation, or as they put it themselves, 'with the greatest possible apprehension'.

> Gynaecological care may be, and in some other countries
> is, interpreted to include provisions for birth limitation
> and abortion. We have no guarantee that State officials
> will respect Catholic principles in regard to these matters.

Again, there is the pejorative reference to 'state officials'. The
hysteria is whipped up in the most cynical fashion. The country
is about to be plunged into a tyrannical nightmare exhibiting all
the worst imaginings of George Orwell,[73] Aldous Huxley[74] and
Batman.[75] And with mischief, 'birth limitation' is lumped in with
abortion – twin evils of comparable scale. No amount of fire and
brimstone and Redemptorist fulmination, however, has in the
intervening years prevented birth control from becoming the
norm for Catholics and it has dropped off the Episcopal radar.[76]

Many years after *Roe versus Wade*[77] in the United States and
David Steele[78] in Great Britain made indiscriminate abortion
normal it has not come to Ireland. This is not due to any action
of the Catholic Hierarchy of 1950 who are roundly ignored
on their twin issue of birth control: it is due to the attitude of
the people. The people for half a century have prised apart the
issues of 'birth limitation and abortion'; the Bishops would have
done better not to have joined them.

> Doctors trained in institutions in which we have no
> confidence may be appointed as medical officers under
> the proposed services, and may give gynaecological care
> not in accordance with Catholic principles.

One has little difficulty in reaching the conclusion that
'institutions in which we have no confidence' are represented *par
excellence* by that academy detested by the Archbishop, Trinity
College. There is also a depressing narrowness to this analysis
which suggests that doctors who might have adventured abroad
to train in more liberal institutions might be compromised
rather than improved by such exposure.

In other Irish universities the Medical Ethics course was often badly taught within the narrow parameters of 'Catholic principles', on occasion by a clergyman of that persuasion. In the author's case a course which should have been probing and philosophical was boring and received by the students with contempt. The examination sanction was brought to bear to stifle any independent interpretation. Any student who, in his answer, struck out on a line which was 'not in accord with Catholic principles' was unceremoniously failed. The lesson of having to return early to repeat his examination in the autumn quickly brought him to heel and by September he was ready to regurgitate stuff which he did not believe, but would pass him. Furthermore, those who came after such a maverick learned this lesson well and regurgitation – as with much else in Ireland at the time – became the norm.

The Irish Medical Association had repeatedly stated the fundamental and entirely reasonable principle that in any new structure 'the doctor-patient relationship must be preserved'. Behind the scenes they succeeded in convincing the Hierarchy that this fundamental relationship was in mortal danger. It is difficult to convince oneself that the senior doctors believed this to be the case, but their objective was achieved: the Bishops were now in full campaign mode in the fight to prevent this imaginary impending apocalypse.

> The proposed service also destroys the confidential relationship between doctor and patient and regards all cases of illness as matter for public records and research without regard to the individual's right to privacy.

To all ethical practitioners of medicine the relationship between doctor and patient, handed down to us since Hippocrates, is sacrosanct. All transactions within that relationship must be guarded with the iron confidentiality of the confessional. Any failure of or threat of intrusion into that confidentiality would render the relationship unworkable, to the detriment of the patient. Nothing must ever be done, or no new structures can be introduced, which might cause any erosion of patient confidence in that relationship. This latter stricture is a powerful and much travelled argument for the maintenance of the status quo. Therein lies the rub.

Why the one-to-one doctor-patient relationship should be compromised by the provision of public rather than private healthcare is not made clear by those who vehemently oppose the former. Indeed, the implied suggestion, by both the Bishops and the Irish Medical Association, that doctors would behave differently with regard to such a fundamental matter, depending on the source of their payment, tends to undermine somewhat their credibility and high moral tone. There is nothing wrong with talking about money up front: everybody deserves a living. To be thinking about money, however, while piously affecting concern for the principles of Hippocrates, is an abuse of the great man.

That is convenient belief.

The obstetrical speciality, of all others, had and has a conspicuous, honourable and long-standing history of maintaining and making public excellent statistical records – indeed, the kind of national maternal and infant mortality statistics which the Minister published in his booklet as the *raison d'être* for his scheme, and which so infuriated the Archbishop. Never has this practice infringed on any patient's rights or confidentiality. On the contrary, countless mothers have been saved from death, and infants from damage, by the epidemiological analysis of such records stigmatised by the Hierarchy of 1950 as 'public'. Ironically, a later Archbishop of Dublin, Diarmuid Martin, stating that Ireland is one of the safest places in the world to have a baby, used these same statistics calmly and convincingly, in his adroit argument against the introduction of abortion.[79] The Catholic regime of 1950, however, characterised these data as 'public records', the word 'public' having decidedly ideological and pejorative undertones.

It is not as though doctors never divulge information about their patients. In fact the routine divulging of masses of information is necessary for the running of society and is mandated under the law. Many infectious diseases, indeed socially embarrassing ones, are reportable. Doctors do not baulk; indeed, they may collect a fee for such reporting. The greater good is served. Neither do they recoil from full medical disclosure, notwithstanding that it may adversely affect their patient's prospects, to insurance companies, potential employers, adoption agencies and a plethora of other bodies both public and private.

To suggest that a publicly funded medical consultation is likely to result in more disclosure than a privately funded one, or as the Bishop of Ferns put it with some hyperbole, more likely to become a 'matter for public records', is absurd. Is there less intrusion by extraneous bodies into patients' affairs in the United States where medicine is predominantly private? Is there more in Britain where it is predominantly public? Indeed, one might expect the opposite to be the case for the following reasons.

Private capital is paying for one and the public purse for the other. When private funders are paying they are not so readily separated from their funds. Private healthcare capitalists protect their profits by minimising risk. Towards this end they collect masses of intrusive data about patients and indeed about whole tranches of the population – and on occasion by dubious means. Better to winnow out the patient who is likely to cost you or your shareholders a lot of money and avoid him: leave his healthcare to the public purse. Indeed such private healthcare funders cannot wait to get their hands on genetic databases in order to avoid, or excessively load, citizens programmed by their DNA to make heavy demands on medical services. In this milieu of private healthcare funding the doctor comes under more pressure than in publicly funded systems for disclosure, which may be detrimental to the patient's interests.

Meanwhile, in publicly funded healthcare systems the politician is in charge. In the auction for votes the politician who presents himself as a health funding Scrooge is likely to experience a short shelf life. He benefits, however, from a confusion in the public mind – particularly among those who pay at the lower end of the tax scale – as to where Government money comes from. While the shareholder knows that the company is spending his money, many a citizen believes that the Government is spending not his but its own money. Regardless of these nuances, however, the politician has the delicious pleasure of always spending other people's money and in the auction for votes, with regard to the provision of health services, he spends it like a drunken sailor.

The provider of universal publicly funded healthcare – that which the IMA described as a 'cancer' and which the Bishop of Ferns said would destroy 'the individual's right to privacy' – does not demand information about your medical history, your genes or your bad habits before taking you on. Indeed, the public provider's behaviour in this regard is in marked contrast to the prescriptive information demands of the private sector: demands for information often made of doctors.

The politician, instead of collecting personal information to isolate vulnerable groups as private entities would do, often responds to the emotional appeal of such groups, and by this populist device harvests a large number of votes. For doctors or Bishops, or indeed Archbishops or anybody else, to insist that State participation in health services intrudes into the doctor-patient relationship is disingenuous at best and at worst downright dishonest.

Rather, it is the case that public healthcare systems, spending as they do only other people's money, intrude less into the hallowed relationship between doctor and patient.

The issue of clinical independence, a tired old canard, is often twinned with that of medical confidentiality in the spurious arguments advanced by those who, for reasons of ideology or venality, argue against the provision of publicly funded healthcare. In the period we are discussing, the gestation and delivery into the world of the British National Health Service found little favour with the medical establishment. In a review of that period published in 1998 entitled '1948: A Turbulent Gestation for the NHS,'[80] the author states, 'only a minority of doctors supported the idea of a state funded health service in 1945'.

Foremost among the objections piously advanced by the British Medical Association (BMA) was the perceived threat to clinical freedom – notwithstanding that most historians consider matters of money to have been uppermost in the organisation's collective mind. Clinical independence (or clinical freedom as it was often called then) was much touted as it would be in Ireland as the Church-Medical alliance, with even greater piety, ramped up its campaign to destroy the Mother and Child Scheme in 1950. The British, however, with their natural reserve avoided the vulgar hyperbole of the Bishop of Ferns, and in any case the Archbishop of Canterbury was publicly in favour of the British scheme.

Doctors, having enjoyed the privilege from ancient times, jealously guard their clinical independence – and so they should. Like all privileges, however, this one has to be earned, cherished and not abused. To abuse it is to risk losing it. The scope of this privilege is open to subjective interpretation. To the thinking man or woman it means the entitlement to do that which is right and reasonable. To a less cerebral colleague it may mean the right to do what is convenient and comfortable. This latter one is frequently to be heard trenchantly defending clinical freedom while at the same time practising in a manner which might not stand up to scrutiny.

In Ireland it is ironic that the Bishops should have advanced themselves as the defenders of clinical freedom. It was they, rather than those pejoratively labelled as 'lay bureaucrats' by the IMA, who intruded into clinical freedom with a list of procedures and practices related to obstetrics, gynaecology and reproduction generally that were denied to patients. Their success in fusing Church and State, in controlling most hospitals directly or vicariously and imposing their will on supine politicians and a beholden medical leadership, resulted in the imposition of this regime upon the entire nation and on those of all faiths or none.

Church-owned private hospitals, accepting no public funds, are perfectly entitled to impose this restriction on clinical freedom; indeed, this represents no more than an admirable adherence to their principles. Other Church-owned hospitals, however, while accepting large tranches of public money, were expected to do likewise as were secular public hospitals funded fully by the taxpayer. The Church enjoyed 'representation without taxation'[81] – a free lunch.

This writer is happy to state that never once during a long career in a public statutory hospital did any 'lay bureaucrat' attempt to interfere with his judgement as to precisely what surgical procedure he might perform for an individual patient. He cannot, however, say the same of the religious community in the same institution. A vignette will serve to make the point.

Occasionally a patient will ask that a sterilisation procedure, which might easily be anatomically incorporated into the bigger primary operation, be added. On one such occasion, as late as 1990, the operating list was prepared and sent to the operating theatre on the day before the planned procedure, as is usual, to enable careful preparation. The precise procedure to be done was stated in its entirety. Not one but two chaplains asked to see the surgeon immediately and came to his office. In so doing they were honourably discharging what they had been trained to consider their duty. Their position was that the operation was immoral, was taking place in a Catholic hospital and must not go ahead. The surgeon's position was that the procedure was perfectly moral and legal, was taking place in a citizen's and not a Church hospital, and would go ahead, with any conscientious objectors (of whom there proved to be none) given the opportunity of absenting themselves from the event. The encounter was civil but there was no meeting of minds. The procedure went ahead with a happy patient unaware of the attempted interference with clinical freedom and confidentiality. Wiser counsel prevailed on the clerical side and the surgeon did not again experience such interference or abuses of patient confidentiality in similar scenarios presenting thereafter.

Such pressure – indeed today it might be called bullying – was commonplace and the medical profession might, with more honour, have been less compliant.

The argument, then, that public medicine would be a great threat to clinical independence was spurious and dishonest. It was advanced by the medical leadership for its own purposes and the Church leadership would better have served its followers by being less credulous. Their credulity however was born of convenience and was conducive to the preservation of their power and influence.

A lie had been defined in the Catholic Catechism for generations of Irish schoolchildren as 'the deliberate intention to deceive'. Their Lordships are engaging in that for which they were teaching children that they would go to Hell.

Having embarked on the process of deception, it was necessary, according to the axiom of the recently departed Herr Goebbels, to tell the lie big. And what could be bigger than that 'all cases of illness' would be exposed to the vulgar gaze. And who bigger to warn of the impending Orwellian nightmare than the Catholic Church? The Hierarchy were not just warning that the new order, for so they were portraying it, would be prone to the occasional medical indiscretion; rather, they were saying that every intimate detail of a patient's afflictions would be laid bare 'as a matter for public records'.

The word 'research' as applied here is used in a negative sense and is calculated to cause the greatest alarm. Their Lordships placed themselves in the category that would later become known as conspiracy theorists. It was not made clear that every state has the right and indeed the duty to collect statistics upon which to plan its health programmes. This legitimate activity is portrayed as a gross invasion of privacy. Doctors have a duty to contribute to the advancement of the science of medicine. The medical leadership should therefore have made it clear that it is possible to collect and interpret indispensable epidemiological information on health and disease without in any way violating 'the individual's right to privacy'. They conspicuously held back, however, from any reassurance regarding that unfounded anxiety.

Any protestation against the view that the Church was being used as a mouthpiece for Medicine must surely be neutered by reading the following:

> The elimination of private medical practitioners by a State-paid service has not been shown to be necessary or even advantageous to the patient, the public in general or the medical profession.

The art of the 'spin doctor' and lobbyist was poorly developed in Ireland in 1950. A nation out through the seat of its trousers offered scant pickings to this parasitic species, which was later to become ubiquitous. The medical establishment, however, in its campaign to destroy the hated Minister for Health and his much misrepresented scheme, had no need to hire such expertise. The purpose of all alliances is, after all, to accomplish together that which might not be possible on one's own. The medical establishment had long since concluded that, on their own, their renegade Minister would get the better of them.

Now, however, they had at their service, gratis, the best public relations apparatus in the land.

Their Lordships, in communicating their messages to the public, enjoyed over public relations consultants one singular advantage then – everybody believed them. This level of credibility was underpinned by more than a hint of infallibility rubbing off their boss in Rome. It is likely, indeed, that the incumbent in Rome, a man of extremely conservative outlook not loved by history, took more than a passing interest in the on-going spat between Church, State and medicine in Ireland. Irish taxpayers, notwithstanding that the country was impoverished, maintained not one but two full embassies in the Eternal City. Of these two legations the lesser was to the nation state of Italy; most of the action was at the more lively station over at the Vatican.[82]

Such were the forces ranged against the hapless Minister in his efforts to save mothers and babies and put shoes on the 'Echo Boy'.

The Hierarchy now lapse into the most transparent advocacy for powerful worldly vested interests in medicine. Unashamedly, they nail their colours to the mast of 'private medical practitioners'. How inappropriate it seems that they should lavish their concern on those at the more opulent end of society in least need of their support. To any dispassionate observer, and indeed to many thoughtful members of the rank and file clergy, it must have appeared discouraging that the Church leadership had strayed so far from the path of the founder of Christianity. The Biblical parable was good opium for the masses, but in their dispute with the Minister the Bishops were on the side of Dives.

For His Lordship of Ferns to try to put it over that the proposed Mother and Child Health Service would not be 'advantageous to the patient' must surely cross the bounds of mendacity. For the Bishops to have believed this would have required them to abandon themselves entirely to self-deception. An alternative and less kindly analysis might be that Their Lordships, in their parallel universe, were entirely detached or, worse still, did not care. It is likely, however, that they did care – Noël Browne makes honourable mention of Bishop Dignan of Clonfert in this regard – but cared more about their powerful position and the threat of its erosion by the upstart Minister.

The statement that the proposed new service would not be 'advantageous to the public in general' rings equally hollow. While it might seem ungracious to conclude that their Lordships were lying, it is nevertheless the case that they were telling the exact opposite of the truth.

Why should Bishops become frenzied as to what was or was not 'advantageous to the medical profession'? Interfering with the perks and privileges of doctors is scarcely a reserved sin[83] requiring the attention of Bishops. What does the word 'advantageous', as used here, mean? 'Advantageous' to medicine might generally be taken as supportive to the science and practice by providing better facilities and structures and more effective treatments. This was, however, precisely what the Minister was proposing. Advantageous to medicine means advantageous to patients.

The Bishops, however, were concerned about what might or might not be 'advantageous to the medical profession' – a different matter entirely. Indeed, one could have a proposal, and there have been many such, which might be advantageous to the art and science of medicine, while at the same time perceived as materially disadvantageous to their interests by the 'medical profession'. Such a proposal, the doctors believed, was precisely what the Minister had on the table.

Medicine in 1950 was, and to a considerable degree remains, a conservative profession. There is nothing wrong with that. A person after all may embrace whichever end of the political spectrum that takes his fancy. He may, furthermore, gravitate towards that end which not only takes his fancy but also suits his purpose. The Minister's scheme did not suit the doyens' purpose for two reasons – money and independence.

Of money in Ireland in 1950 there was very little. Of that little bit that was available however the doctors, and particularly the senior urban medical cognoscenti, got more than a fair share. This position was felt to be well worth defending. And the medical establishment in Ireland has always been a stout defender of its interests. When allied with the Catholic Hierarchy, however, even when their arguments were transparently bogus and flew in the face of both Hippocrates and Jesus Christ, the doyens of medicine were more than a match for the Minister with whom they had joined battle.

The idea of working for the State for a salary and be considered a mere public servant was alien to the mindset of the typical doyen of medicine. There was, indeed, a certain contempt for what they considered the token resistance which the British medical establishment had offered before accepting that status under the new National Health Service. There were, however, profound cultural differences. The tradition of public service had been forged in Britain by centuries of empire. In Ireland the behaviour of that same empire had the opposite effect. Successful doctors, along with their Episcopal allies, used this suspicion of central authority as a rationale for keeping the State out of medicine.

Altogether more germane to the doctors' thinking, however, was probably their idea that 'State paid' would be badly paid. The State had, after all, been governed since independence by an admirably ascetic and idealistic breed of revolutionary politicians who were very tight on the purse strings. The doctors had no confidence that State largesse would be lavished on them with any more abandon than it was on poorly paid teachers, police, civil servants and many others. There were, however, probably many doctors who were far from rich and would welcome the status of being 'State paid'. It was not, however, for those that the top dogs in medicine or their friends in the Hierarchy spoke.

Bad though it would be to be 'State paid' the scenario outlined for the doctors by the Bishop of Ferns was much worse. Using unrestrained language 'private medical practitioners' would, according to him suffer 'elimination'. This was, of course, never going to happen and Their Lordships must have known it. They were disingenuously intimating that the scheme would be, or would become, compulsory. The Minister had, however, stated, in the clearest terms and repeatedly, that participation by patients and doctors would be voluntary. People would have been at liberty to take or leave the new service. Those in most need would obviously take it while the more comfortable would be at liberty to make their own arrangements and pay 'private medical practitioners'.

The scenario disingenuously outlined by the Bishop of Ferns – the elimination of private medical practitioners – filled the doyens with foreboding. A reliable stream of income, and indeed a poorly documented one, might completely disappear. True, the State might, as had happened with Britain's National Health Service, pay the doctors well at the start to rope them in, but the honeymoon would soon be over. As Government and doctors settled down to the humdrum of life together, the latter believed that, at least with regard to matters of money, they would be unhappy bedfellows. Shotgun weddings – for such was this union to be – do not make for domestic bliss.

The doctors probably believed that, even if their campaign to frustrate the Minister, with its many meetings and poll of members around the country, failed, significant private practice would, as discussed above, remain. There was, however, an alternative and altogether more alarming scenario menacing the 'private medical practitioners'.

Suppose, perish the thought, that the Minister's scheme became a runaway success. Noël Browne, for all his angularity, had a reputation for getting things done and had already, with modest resources, accomplished much. Suppose he brought this same efficiency to bear on his Mother and Child Health Service, and all those eligible began voting with their feet to avail of the new service for which his Lordship of Ferns had expressed such lofty contempt.

The effect of this Ministerial success would be twofold: a marked improvement in the health and safety of mothers and children and a marked disimprovement, although difficult to quantify, in the income of certain doyen doctors. This was something up with which the latter were not prepared to put. This fault line between what is in the best interest of medicine and what is in the best interest of 'medical practitioners' was, for those who wished to see it, cruelly exposed by the Mother and Child debacle, and has bedevilled the structure of Irish healthcare ever since.

Independence is an admirable trait and doctors could, like everybody else, be expected to protect theirs. They were, however, more than a little disingenuous in the extent to which they were protesting in negotiations that their independence was threatened. History has shown that doctors, like all other groups, were never affronted by being 'State paid' when the State pay was right. Independence however was a great card to play to cement the Episco-Medical alliance.

As long as the doctors remained 'independent' the Hierarchy were confident that they would do their bidding and Their Lordships' writ would run. A medical profession independent of the State would be sound on issues of 'faith and morals'. This, however, was an extremely qualified form of independence and there must have been some who would have preferred the indignity of being 'State paid' to that of being crozier-whipped, and being completely submissive to Drumcondra.

The Bishop of Ferns now, having got the big stuff off his chest, seeks to portray the position of the Hierarchy as sweet reasonableness.

> The Bishops are most favourable to measures which would benefit public health, but they consider that instead of imposing a costly bureaucratic scheme of nationalised medical service the State might well consider the advisability of providing the maternity hospitals and other institutional facilities which are at the present lacking and should give adequate maternity benefits and taxation relief for large families.

This passage is unctuous and condescending in the extreme.

Their Lordships' words and particularly their actions are far from convincing that, particularly with regard to mothers and children, they are preoccupied by a desire to 'benefit public health'. On the contrary, one might reasonably conclude that their agitation related to matters of private healthcare rather than improving the 'public health'. How could anybody be other than 'favourable to any measures that would benefit public health'? Yet their Lordships, the most powerful moral force in the land, feel obliged to reassure us that they are just that. Their reassurances make the Hierarchy seem less sure footed. Is it possible that, unconvinced of the rectitude of the position which they have adopted, they 'doth protest too much'. It is worth reflecting that the public health problems which the Minister was trying to confront were of the most urgent life and death kind, and the best device which the Bishops could muster to block him was to insist that his new programme would not be free for all and must be restricted by a means test.

Following Bishop Staunton's opening gambit that the Hierarchy is 'most favourable to measures which would benefit the public health', he enters a series of caveats which compromise his sincerity and which, if applied, would hobble the Minister's scheme entirely.

The Hierarchy, they would have us believe, were in favour of the scheme, in principle. Those who toil interminably at health service meetings today will know what this perversion of English means – they were against it.

The truth, as it appears in the cold light of the twenty-first century, is that Dr Noël Browne, as Minister for Health, was trying to accomplish by political measures that which should have been the concern of both medicine and Church and in which both were delinquent – improvement in the lot of the most wretched in society. This surely should have been the ambition of the Church-medical alliance but, in a reversal of what should have been their roles, they engaged in an unholy and un-Hippocratic conspiracy to prevent this progress.

It is not perhaps surprising that organised medicine should try to preserve its material interests: most groups would do the same. For the Hierarchy, however, to affect concern for the poor while at the same time resisting measures which would improve their lot was less than edifying.

Having reassured the Taoiseach that, notwithstanding all their words and actions to the contrary, the Hierarchy are in favour of 'measures which would benefit public health', their scribe the Bishop of Ferns now turns his attention to the matter of 'costly bureaucracy'.

Costly Bureaucracy

The analysis of bureaucracy, particularly by populist journalism, of the Irish Health Service has always been superficial. Entirely essential support grades, for example clinical secretaries, medical records staff, receptionists and many others who deal daily with patient's problems, and who exist in great numbers and are not highly paid, are classified as 'administration' – bureaucracy.

It is safe ground to condemn bureaucracy, particularly when it is 'costly' – indeed, what other kind of bureaucracy is there? It has in fact since become clear, with regard to healthcare in

Ireland and elsewhere, that you can have a big health service with much bureaucracy, you can have a small health service with almost as much bureaucracy, but what you cannot have is any health service at all without bureaucracy. Their Lordships would have known this. They themselves were, after all, for two millennia the great exponents of the bureaucratic art. Here however 'Ferns' resorts to the ploy of using the word pejoratively and with much ingenuity. He is writing to the Taoiseach, the head of Government, over the head of the Minister for Health and is undermining the latter. When Bishops in 1950 began to undermine, collapse of the edifice became inevitable.

It always pleases a head of Government to be told of ways in which money can be saved. It is doubly pleasing to be cautioned in advance of impending 'costly bureaucratic schemes'. The Bishops are in effect counselling the Taoiseach to use cost as an excuse for abandoning the scheme (and the Minister). If such a scheme were to be received with universal acclaim and Episcopal approbation it would, regardless of the cost, be politically attractive and the Taoiseach would jump at it. The Minister's scheme however enjoyed none of these attributes but rather came with a string of potentially toxic complications.

Having undermined the Minister's scheme by describing it as 'costly and bureaucratic', 'Ferns' lands the killer blow: the scheme is, in addition, to be that most detestable of all inventions, 'a scheme of nationalised medical service'.

It is clear that Their Lordships, while probably having little experience of the nationalised health services available for scrutiny elsewhere, regarded such arrangements as having been contrived by the devil himself. Furthermore, such schemes were predominantly to be found in countries of Northern Europe and indeed mainly in those of the Protestant tradition.

The old *bête noir* Great Britain, along with the Scandinavian countries, were prime exemplars of this iniquity. Sweden in particular, using this model of 'nationalised' healthcare, could produce extremely relevant statistics on such parameters as maternal and infant mortality, infectious disease, life expectancy and many others that were the envy of the world. The Swedes were also of course, with regard to their prevailing sexual mores, famously ahead of the time and this aspect of their society aroused much outside curiosity not least in Ireland. The Irish Bishops, in their self-appointed role as custodians of the nation's morals, were ever on guard against the introduction of licentious behaviour commonplace in such alien countries.

The highly successful Scandinavian model of healthcare was damned by its association with liberated sexual behaviour portrayed by its film industry. Such twin evils had no place in Catholic Ireland. The film censor, who was also under the joyless boot of Drumcondra, would keep out the dirty movies and his Grace and Their Lordships would keep out the equally odious 'nationalised medical service'.

Yet again Their Lordships have turned logic on its head. While professing themselves in favour of 'any measures that would benefit public health', they seek to obstruct the Minister from introducing much needed measures which would do just that. Their attitude is in tune, not with orderly regimes in Northern Europe which looked after their citizens well, but rather with the neglectful Romance countries of Southern Europe – the chaos of Italy along with the unsavoury regimes of Franco in Spain and Salazar in Portugal. These latter, of course, spared their citizens the evils that 'nationalised medical service' would bring.

The Hierarchy, having made it plain to the Taoiseach that the Mother and Child Scheme was not acceptable to them, now offer their own prescription for the health of the nation. This passage of the letter is extraordinary in that it proposes much of what the Minister had in mind anyway or has already accomplished. The Hierarchy, however, offers this wisdom as if it were the fruit of their own deliberations, a ploy to which during the dispute they frequently resorted.

Their Lordships are trying to steal the Minister's clothes while they insist that he don the means test garment.

The Ferns letter to the Taoiseach concludes with, if we may borrow a term from Islam, an Episcopal fatwa.[84]

> The Bishops desire that your Government should give careful consideration to the dangers inherent in the present proposals before they are adopted by the Government for legislative enactment and therefore they feel it their duty to submit their views on this subject to you privately and at the earliest opportunity, since they regard the issues involved as of the gravest moral and religious importance.

This, the concluding paragraph of the letter, is dripping with menace. Readers two-thirds of a century later may not perceive the passage as menacing: they may indeed find much of it quite reasonable. He is, however, not for the first time in his letter, resorting to an artful combination of intimidation and reasonableness.

First the intimidation.

The diminishing band of those who were alive and aware in 1950 will understand how impolitic it would have been for the Government, or anybody else, to ignore what 'the Bishops desire'. Their Lordships were, of course, perfectly entitled to desire whatsoever they pleased and indeed to express their views. They were not, however, entitled to intimidate the Government with the innuendo that they could and would bring it down (as subsequently happened). Up until now the exercise of 'soft power' – simply indicating their 'desire' – had usually served to induce political compliance. It had usually been sufficient for their gunboat to loiter demonstratively. Now however its guns were locked and loaded and trained on the Minister and the entire Government. The phoney war was over.

To give 'careful consideration' to new departures is of course the wisest of advice. Such advice, however, emanating from Their

Catholic Lordships and committed to paper by their secretary, emphasising 'the dangers inherent in the present proposals', was a clear statement of intent. Danger meant danger to the Government, the elected Government. The Hierarchy were in effect saying to the head of Government, we call the shots. They were saying you are in office on sufferance, our sufferance, and if you do not do our bidding we will rouse the country against you and your Government will fall.

Next the reasonableness.

Nobody would dispute their Lordships' right, or perhaps even their duty as Staunton put it, 'to submit their views on this subject', or indeed any other. The Bishops in addition affected a most tender concern for the sensitivities of the Government – they were submitting their views 'privately'. There was really no need for the citizens to be made privy to the efforts of the Hierarchy to spare them the rigours of an improved health service. And furthermore, what could be more reasonable than putting the Taoiseach on notice of the 'dangers inherent' in the troublesome Minister's scheme at 'the earliest opportunity'. It is in his closing words that Staunton reaches his most surreal heights of absurdity – 'the issues involved are of the gravest moral and religious importance'. It is worth reflecting briefly on what were 'the issues involved' because by now they had become completely lost in the fog of war.

Firstly, 'the rights of the family' must be preserved – entirely reasonable. In this instance, however, it meant preserving their right, especially those at the lower end of the socio-economic spectrum, to endure continuing medical neglect and all the other social and biological evils attendant upon poverty. Also involved was the right to be spared 'totalitarian aggression'. For the State to look after its most wretched citizens amounted, by this cold war innuendo, to communism.

A further great evil was that the State proposed to make 'social policy' for 'the whole community'. This their Lordships considered to be their own prerogative. It would appear that the Minister's proposal, if 'adopted by the Government for legislative enactment', would, by looking after the health of mothers and children, cause the country to sink into a miasma of depravity and perdition. In addition, doctors who were 'State paid' would be incapable of patient confidentiality. The State would, of course, direct reproductive behaviour: abortion would be in, euthanasia would follow. All of these and many other abominations which would flow from the provision of improved mother and child health services would destroy the Catholic moral virtue of the nation.

These many impending evils presented the Episcopal custodians of the nation's soul with a very great problem indeed. They did, however, recognise their responsibility and devoted themselves energetically to finding a solution. On many occasions they foregathered at the fountain of their formation at Maynooth in search of the wisdom which would save the nation. These men, often academically brilliant but somewhat de-intellectualised by the stultifying and institutionally narcissistic process of their higher education, would not be found wanting and sure enough the solution materialised. With the tailwind of divine inspiration the solution when it came, as is often the case, was simple.

The people, apart from the 'necessitous' 10 per cent, must be made to pay for the service and thus would all the moral hazard be removed.

This simple device would be a panacea. The danger of communism, and we should remember that in 1950 the Russians were at the gates, would be averted. The lower orders of society would receive a clear signal as to their place in the scheme of things and they would know their place – they belonged to the 'necessitous 10 per cent'. If only the Mother and Child Service could be means tested it would, as if by magic, no longer be 'subject to very great abuse'. In addition, means testing would remove anxiety about 'important moral questions' – as to precisely how it would accomplish this is not made clear. Not least amongst the potential benefits of means testing would be the salvation of 'Catholic girls and women' from perdition at the hands of 'State paid' doctors, particularly such doctors as were trained in educational institutions in which Their Lordships had 'no confidence'.

There was one other extraordinary effect which a means test, so beloved by McQuaid and the Hierarchy, would have: it related to their lack of affection for 'bureaucracy'.

Those familiar with the Irish healthcare system, then and now, know that, while it has many failings, the system excels in one regard – it does bureaucracy well. When any new task appears, and the implementation of a means test for every family in the land would be no small task, it cannot be discharged by existing incumbents. Restrictive practices mandate the hiring of extra operatives for the new function. The numbers required to assess the means of so many citizens would be very great indeed and might, humbler folk could be tempted to believe, greatly increase rather than diminish 'expensive bureaucracy'.

In effect, the elimination of a means test, as proposed by the Minister, would mean less, not more, bureaucracy.

The Bishop of Ferns had, with some absurdity, manoeuvred himself into a position of *non sequitur*. Clearly these two positions, that of what we are calling ordinary folk and of Their Lordships, were not reconcilable. A robust body politic might indeed have demanded of Their Lordships some explanation of this contradiction. Notwithstanding their affectation of Parliamentary Democracy, however, in the view of the craven Government of the time, the opinions of ordinary folk stacked up poorly against those of Bishops. In any case, when Bishops insisted that something was so, regardless of its absurdity, that was that. Bishops, when they spoke *una voce*, did not do explanation.

7

The Lines are Drawn

Thus by mid-twentieth century the battle lines to determine the future structure and direction of the Irish health service were drawn. All that was required to set off the conflagration was a Sarajevo moment. History obliged by throwing up a concordance of personalities and circumstances which could not have been better contrived to produce combustion. The battle would be fought on ground carefully chosen by one of the antagonists, the Archbishop of Dublin, but disastrously blundered into by the other, the Minister for Health.

By 1950 in Ireland the art of delivering babies was well worked out but poorly catered for. Obstetrics and midwifery, to their credit, were and remain one of the few areas of medicine to collect and indeed publish reliable statistics of outcomes. These statistics, notwithstanding the work of some notable institutions, revealed a deplorable situation. Such poor outcomes were due as much to social deprivation and its many attendant miseries as to the deficiencies of medical knowledge. While the requisite medical knowledge existed, medical services were poorly developed and organised, and to the extent that they existed at all, they were available mainly to those in least need of them – the better off. For the majority, pregnancy looked after itself. There might or might not be some help with the mechanical act of delivery, often provided by unregulated 'handy women', but thereafter the patients were sent on their way. The regime was one of ad hoc and crisis management.

While this regime obtained throughout the whole of medicine at that time, end points in obstetrics are defined by a stark clarity: a dead or live mother, a dead or live baby, a baby whole or maimed. Some of these disasters are, of course, at any time and in all societies unavoidable. Many, however, can be prevented or attenuated by extending care throughout pregnancy, through delivery and into its aftermath – precisely what Dr Noël Browne, Minister for Health was proposing.

STREPTOMYCIN AND BISHOPS

Politicians like to do big things, to leave their mark, and so it was with the Minister for Health of 1950, Noël Browne, who was already widely acclaimed for his success – mainly due to the serendipitous arrival of new drugs, particularly streptomycin, and good organisational structures – in tackling the national scourge of tuberculosis. He now proposed to use his office to introduce a completely free scheme to improve the deplorable lot of mothers and children.

The Minister might have anticipated that the former task – the *tubercle bacillus* was after all one of the great historic curses of humanity – would have been the more difficult. Furthermore, the improvement of services for mothers and children was more a matter of organisation and structure than of advanced science. His anticipation of the relative difficulty of the two tasks, however, was confounded by two variables, one new, the other ancient.

We refer respectively to streptomycin and the Bishops.

That it should prove easier to banish epidemic tuberculosis than to institute a much needed programme of care for mothers and their children runs counter to all rational intuition, but such is what came to pass.

The Minister in question, certainly something of a maverick and a man with whom it was not difficult to disagree,[85] was, as with many who have held that portfolio, trained as a medical doctor. This equipped him with a penetrating insight into the foibles of his own kind and the chafing interface between medicine and politics. His erudition, intellectual mien and somewhat supercilious manner set him apart from the common run of earthy politicians.[86] In addition, he was a member of a minor leftish political party,[87] the junior partners in a somewhat fractious coalition Government. These points are made not in any way to detract from the man's credibility but rather to emphasise his vulnerability. In fact his credibility, integrity and reputation generally have been fortified with every passing year of the intervening six decades. He was, however, in the Ireland of his time something of a political outsider functioning in a glasshouse – a dangerous place to throw stones.

The stone which the Minister threw, immortalised in Irish medical, political and ecclesiastical folklore, was that which has become synonymous with his name – the Mother and Child Scheme.

The Mother and Child Scheme, designed, as its naming suggests, to support all mothers, regardless of their means, during and after pregnancy and their children up to the age of 16 years, must have seemed, to most observers, unpromising material for controversy. The service would be free, universally available and provided as of right by the State. There would be no means test. Everybody was to be a winner – or so one might think.

The Irish Medical Association, however, hated the plan and set about its destruction. To devise an undermining strategy, however, while at the same time posturing to remain in favour of the aims of such a worthy and popular measure, was no easy task. To this end the antagonists fell back on two old reliables, doublethink and the Bishops.

It should be remembered that the period under discussion was that of Josef Stalin, Joseph McCarthy and Castelgandolfo.

In the modern epoch the prevailing atmosphere with regard to Church and State finds its closest echo in Iran at the start of the twenty-first century. In the Ireland of mid-twentieth century, however, the concept of 'the Supreme Religious Leader' was already well developed. He, Archbishop John Charles McQuaid, governed from Drumcondra – from a 'palace'.

The Supreme Leader, unelected though he was, wielded great power in this 'Republic'. Any legislation or measure which might impinge on his wide ranging prerogatives had first to be submitted for approval, or indeed veto, to the incumbent of the said palace. Such approval could by no means be taken for granted. It was not at all as cut and dried as when, for example, a British Prime Minister went to the palace. Elected British politicians, in a constitutional monarchy, as a matter of courtesy, informed the palace of what was to be done. Elected Irish politicians, in a Republic, got clearance from the palace as to what was allowed to be done. The irony of this situation was lost on most citizens.

The Minister had a good reputation for getting things done. There is little doubt that his Mother and Child proposal would further have fortified his standing. The forces of reaction however – favourite verbiage of Moscow at the time – were afoot.

While the Mother and Child Scheme will forever be associated with Noël Browne and the first coalition Government of John A. Costello, it is less appreciated that it was conceived and legislated for in 1947 by the previous Fianna Fáil Government under de Valera. That Government had backed off the implementation of the scheme in the face of episcopal opposition. The Archbishop might reasonably have assumed that he would likewise prevail with the present Government. He would, however, find the present incumbent of the Department of Health less tractable.

Also, the proposed scheme would somewhat tread on the toes of the Archbishop's own charitable initiatives to improve the lot of women. Church charity, however, was fair enough – no threat to the fibre of the nation. State interference in such matters, providing services as a right, was a different matter entirely.

Undermining the Minister

The Minister for Health at the same time had great credibility. He had by his achievements, his populist proposal and his transparent idealism, struck a chord with the people. The strategy adopted by the doyens to counter his scheme was ahead of its time. It would be half a century before this strategy was crystallised by the nefarious Carl Rove[88] to achieve the unlikely re-election of George W. Bush as President of the United States: contrary to all intuition and received wisdom, you should attack not your enemy's weaknesses but his strengths.

The Minister's strength was his credibility: it must be undermined.

That the Minister was a graduate of the Archbishop's *bête noir*, Trinity College, must have been tossed early into the mix. To have been nurtured in such a place, and indeed to have ignored His Grace's fatwa on going there, would immediately have rendered him suspect in the eyes of the powerful prelate. It can be assumed in addition that the Minister's medical adversaries would, for the most part, have been graduates of the less ancient arriviste universities catering for the majority religion. The prevailing unseemly intimacy between Church and State penetrated these latter academic institutions to a much greater degree. Graduates of these universities, now in the Archbishop's ear, would have much more credibility – they would be perceived by him as sound. The Minister's enemies were off to a flying start.

The Minister, following his undergraduate education and graduation from an institution in which Their Lordships had 'no confidence', took himself off for postgraduate studies to another place not socially engineered to their taste – England. This migration would have been brought about, as was commonplace, by an ambition to improve himself educationally but also, being unconnected, by necessity. Indeed, it is likely that some of those now engaged in the undermining had been given their jobs under the patronage of His Grace and as a consequence had been spared the rigours of such travel and improvement.

Undoubtedly in that alien place the already suspect medical traveller would have imbibed further dangerous ideas. Had the State there, in the guise of the National Health Service, not taken over medicine completely? The doctors' organisation there, the British Medical Association, had fought it tooth and claw but had been seen off – or indeed as it emerged been bought off[89] – by a determined Government. That the ambitious medical renegade of the left, Dr Noël Browne, should return from such a place, enter politics, get elected at his first attempt and, as a political novice, be appointed as Minister for Health, filled certain elements of the medical establishment with consternation. The job now was to infect, with this consternation, those who could torpedo the Minister and his plan – Their Lordships and their main man in Drumcondra.

There can be little doubt that, in the indoctrination of His Grace, the relative youth of the Minister for Health would have been raised at an early time. The Archbishop, although in his late middle years, had the appearance of a man who was only getting his second wind. The Minister by contrast was little more than half the age of his powerful adversary. He would undoubtedly have been represented by his detractors as callow. This was a dangerous neophyte, intent on imposing alien concepts erosive of the moral fibre of the nation. The role of the Catholic Church, long the custodian of such values, would be usurped by this new State service and by the undoubted panoply of others that would follow.

The Minister, however, was not for turning. He was an acknowledged master of communication and news management. Sound bites like 'no doctor's bills' and 'the people have willed it' were invaluable in the promotion of his project. He was, however, up against stout opposition on the media front. Their Lordships were also masterful in feeding information to a supine press (perhaps with the exception of *The Irish Times*) and to the national broadcaster which was a tame *porte-parole* for the Church's banal views.

But soon there would be more to report than banalities.

Parnell Lurking

The case of Parnell,[90] destroyed by clerical machination half a century before, lived on in the national consciousness. It must indeed have been uppermost in the minds of many around the cabinet table. The ghost of Parnell haunted the Government and the doctors knew it.

They would induce the Hierarchy to 'do a Parnell' on the hapless Minister.

To stoke clerical hysteria about the potential evils of the proposed scheme, the doyens of medicine, through their Association, resorted to much scaremongering, mischief and distortion. The doctor-patient relationship would of course be an early casualty. The business of a State Medical Officer would be the business of the State and, as with all State business, would be a public matter. The great Catholic taboos of contraception, abortion, divorce and euthanasia would become the norm when the State took control. The Minister's Mother and Child Scheme would be the thin end of the wedge that would open the door to a totalitarian state and all its accompanying evils. Were these evils not well exemplified by the excesses of the Nazi regime in Germany still being uncovered? The German example, however – their German Lordships not having distinguished themselves in resisting Hitler – would have played second fiddle to the bogeyman of communism which embodied all the worst fears of the Hierarchy.

The obsession of the Bishops, however, related to matters of faith and morals. In a peculiar Irish idiom of the English language at that time, the word morals in bishopspeak meant one thing only – sexual behaviour. In most societies which acknowledge the Ten Commandments, it is number five which predominates, thou shalt not kill. In twentieth century Ireland, however, it was different – number six was king: thou shalt not commit adultery. And indeed very sound advice it was too, along with the other nine. The point, however, is that Their Lordships had lost their sense of balance. To the detriment of all the social evils proscribed by the other nine they were excessively preoccupied by that forbidden by the sixth – adultery.

The Hierarchy, strangely, seemed to believe that there would be, as a consequence of the proposed legislation, much adultery and moral decay. The precise relationship between better medical services for mothers and their children and worse moral behaviour not however being immediately obvious, there would be further resort to the well tried metaphor of the wedge – and its thin end. It was indeed scarcely necessary to enumerate all the evils that would follow: generic examples would suffice. Ireland would go the way of England. But from the Bishops' perspective there was worse. England, after all, was Protestant. What could you expect? Much more alarming as an example was France where the Reformation had been rejected (the Archbishop of Dublin was a noted Francophile and accomplished French speaker). In France the wedge of secularism had been inserted at a much earlier time and gradually the role of the once powerful Catholic Church, and more to the point its Hierarchy, had been reduced to an irrelevancy. It would happen in Ireland as elsewhere. Once a start had been made on the health service, over time further legislative mallet blows would be struck to drive the secular wedge home. The power of the Church, theretofore the lynchpin of the comfortable status quo in medicine, would be undermined. The country literally and metaphorically would go to hell.

The medical campaign to recruit Their Lordships to the cause was well conceived and orchestrated. It was reminiscent of that, barely ten years before, by which Winston Churchill had induced Franklin Roosevelt to join in the war against Germany and Japan. And now, providentially, Pearl Harbour presented itself in the form of the Minister's iniquitous scheme. The beleaguered doctors, standing alone against the evil Minister and in danger of going under, had succeeded in recruiting to their campaign the greatest power of all, the Church Militant.

The *ad hominem* campaign of whispering, innuendo and malicious rumour against the Minister, already under way, was now ramped up. His true Catholicism was questioned. His 'moral' bona fides were suspect. And all of this in a country where most had not been educated beyond primary level and trusted the Bishops to do their thinking. The people – the voters – took their guidance from the Bishops. The politicians took their signals from the people and perceived a shift in the wind. Perhaps it might be wise to trim their sails accordingly. The rock upon which Parnell had foundered was after all a 'moral' one and now it lurked again. Anything to do with sex and reproduction was quicksand into which Their Militant Lordships could make Ministers and indeed whole Governments disappear.

8

THE NEW RULERS

Ireland in 1950 was a Republic in name only. The captains and the kings of the British Empire had departed but an indigenous elite had moved into the void thus vacated. In this new Republic the religious elite were referred to as the Princes of the Church, and children in schools were conditioned to perceive them as quasi-temporal rulers. Indeed, all the regalia and titles of royalty were retained. The conspicuous obsequiousness of elected politicians in their public display will be remembered today only by a few: their correspondence however is preserved as evidence of total subservience. Furthermore, many who postured at a secular independence were unmasked as, in due course, archival material became available. Letters to Bishops, arch or ordinary, were always prefixed respectfully with titles evocative of temporal power rather than spirituality.

It seems to have been depressing only to a few that a nation which recently, and with violence, had ejected a monarchy and its titled clients, and now styled itself as a Republic, had replaced the *ancien régime* with an indigenous theocratic elite using the same titles and an equal match for their predecessors in pomp and circumstance.

THE MOUNTAIN AND MUHAMMAD

It was natural that a meeting should take place between the primary adversaries in the Mother and Child controversy, the Minister for Health and the Archbishop of Dublin. The Minister was of the expectation, one might think reasonably, that such important Government business with a member of cabinet would take place on State turf, that is, in his department. He was, however, quickly disabused of that notion. He was informed by his departmental secretary that on such occasions established protocol required elected Government Ministers to go to the palace at Drumcondra and play away from home on His Grace's pitch – Muhammad[91] must go to the mountain. Or, as Noël Browne put it in his memoir, 'I was peremptorily ordered to Archbishop McQuaid's palace by a telephone call from his secretary'.

The events surrounding that meeting exemplify yet again, for those who doubt, the master-servant relationship between Church and State in the Ireland of 1950 (and for many years thereafter). While unhappy to sacrifice the principle of the primacy of the State over unelected sectional interests, Noël Browne agreed, in the hope of salvaging his scheme, to travel to the palace for a meeting on the day after the Ferns letter was delivered to the Taoiseach. He was unaware of the existence of the letter and knew nothing of its lethal contents. Notwithstanding that, he was still a devout Catholic and was completely taken aback by the next piece of Episcopal chicanery.

It is a time honoured feature of medical training that all official transactions and professional encounters are contemporaneously and fully documented. The Minister for Health, being a doctor, had been so trained and brought this discipline to his ministry. It was therefore standard practice to take a senior civil servant along to all important meetings in order to document events – simple professionalism. For the meeting at Drumcondra, promising to be of fundamental importance, the Minister decided to take along the Secretary of his department, a man of great experience, integrity, ability and loyalty. The unfortunate Secretary, however, for the second time, had to educate his Minister on the protocol governing such encounters with the Archbishop. Under no circumstances could the Secretary attend. The Minister must come alone. There would be no minutes of the meeting nor any documentation whatsoever. McQuaid was a master of deniability. The *modus operandi* of His Grace was worthy of the Medici and the Borgias of whom he was perhaps an admirer. His control of the venue, the actors and the agenda was complete. The youthful Minister, stripped of the moral and practical support of his experienced departmental Secretary, and deprived of any formal agenda, had no idea in advance of by whom or by how many he might be confronted if he agreed to go to Drumcondra. He was a man of great procedural correctness and was much worried by these Byzantine arrangements. He had furthermore been warned by a political confidant never to go to such important meetings without a witness.

THE MEETING

The account of the meeting (11 October 1950) which survives is that provided by the Minister in his autobiography.[92] He did not write it until a quarter of century had passed. No official minutes are known to exist.

According to his own account, Noël Browne was courteously ushered by the Archbishop into a reception room wherein were gathered two other formidable Princes of the Church.

The first was Dr Michael Browne, Bishop of Galway, a high profile and vociferous martinet whose conservatism was beyond any scale of measurement. The country was well accustomed to hearing his every killjoy utterance regurgitated by the obedient national broadcaster. It is he who is etched in this writer's news-avid childhood memory for an outburst, faithfully relayed on the main evening news one hot summer Sunday, against 'the evils of mixed bathing'. Even a fine summer day in a very capricious climate carried unfathomable potential for evil in the strange mind of this man. The Minister must have found the presence of such a man less than auspicious.

The second personality of the Episcopal triumvirate was none other than the Secretary and scribe to the Hierarchy and the scourge of communists, the Bishop of Ferns, James Staunton. Staunton, although enjoying less notoriety in national reportage than the Bishop of Galway, would later fortify his already adequate bigoted pedigree by his handling of the Fethard on Sea fiasco[93] on his own obscure patch.

It is emblematic of the dysfunction and subservience of the body politic that its Minister for Health, on official business, should have to go alone into the lion's den without the support of his departmental Secretary, while the opposition, the Hierarchy, brought along its Secretary and the diehard Bishop of Galway for good measure.

Into the forbidding ambiance of that drawing room in Drumcondra, peopled by three of the most powerful prelates in the land, the Minister brought a combination of innocence and idealism, rare in politicians, which rendered him poorly equipped to deal with the Byzantine machinations of Their Lordships.

The Minister was the product of a very conventional, indeed Jesuit, early education. This, in spite of his subsequent medical training at Trinity College, left him unable to believe Catholic Bishops capable of such cynicism and of such a cavalier attitude to the health of the poor and of the nation generally, as their behaviour would now indicate. Innocent of the ways of Bishops, he stumbled into their web of intrigue. He was also more innocent than he should have been, given his brains and education, of the capacity of prosperous metropolitan doyen doctors for similar self-serving intrigue.

Having spent many of his most formative years in the English establishment, albeit the *demi-monde* of the English Catholic establishment, he was innocent of the difference between the English and Irish character, the former orderly and obedient, the latter intractable and truculent. He also appears to have been innocent of the common genetic origins of much of the clerical establishment and the doyens of medicine. DNA had not yet been defined[94] but even the most innocent should have known that blood is thicker than water. It is clear that the Minister still carried a great deal of Catholic baggage. To believe that the Bishops were capable of the skulduggery in which they were now engaged would have required him to jettison his faith. That would come later, but for now he was still too innocent to make that radical leap.

Not even the most implacable detractors of Noël Browne can with credibility deny that, for all his many faults, he was an idealist. Idealism is admirable but it is dangerous, particularly in an inflexible personality. Large mature societies, such as Noël Browne had encountered in his youth in England, are more accommodating to the idealist, the individualist, the maverick: the boat is bigger, it is more difficult to rock. The Irish boat in 1950, however, was small indeed and its finely tuned equilibrium, with their Lordships at the helm, was easy to disturb. The arrival of misguided idealism – for such, judged by their behaviour, must have been Their Lordships' view of the Mother and Child Scheme and of State intervention in healthcare matters generally – and of big alien Northern European ideas, had the potential to rock the boat mightily.

Worse still the crew might mutiny and the officers, Their Lordships, in the manner of Captain Bligh,[95] might be consigned to the lifeboats or worse. The fate of many of the Spanish clergy during the civil war had indeed been worse and the Opus Dei[96] version of events was, without balance, indoctrinated into Irish schoolchildren at the time. The Spanish Republic, little more than a dozen years before, while founded in idealism, had resorted to the slaughter of priests. According to the version taught in Ireland, however, Catholic Spain was saved from Godless barbarism by the victory of Catholicism and of Generalissimo Franco.

It is intriguing to ponder whether 'Ferns', true to his calling as scribe to the Hierarchy, might perhaps have recorded the events of the day. The Catholic Church is nothing if not methodical. Is it possible that there exists buried deep in the Dublin Diocesan Archive or elsewhere a document which might clarify events? Certainly the Bishop of Ferns would not be inhibited in his documentation by any threat of disclosure: the impenetrability of Church records is legendary, and has been exemplified many times since.

Accounts of what happened at the meeting between Noël Browne and the assembled Episcopal triumvirate are wildly at variance. It is only fair, since Noël Browne was the only one to favour us with a written account, his autobiography, to give his version of events first.

On entering the room the Minister had read out to him by the Archbishop the full text of the letter (Appendix 1) from Ferns which the Taoiseach had received the previous day, setting out the Hierarchy's rationale for objecting to the Minister's scheme. There followed a discussion in which he attempted to correct what he called some 'false conclusions' they had reached. He felt that the Bishops were excessively concerned about what he called 'temporal issues' rather than spiritual matters, with the Bishop of Galway being particularly exercised on 'the burden of rates and taxation' which would result from the scheme. There was 'a distinct cooling in the previously warm manner of the Archbishop' when he questioned the role of the State in 'the education of mothers in motherhood'. In the face of this the Minister says that he offered concessions.

> I compromised on the offending clauses. In respect of 'the education of mothers', I would reconsider these clauses and submit them to the Hierarchy. Alternatively the Hierarchy could consider the offending clauses

and submit them to the Department of Health for improvement. I was convinced that I had satisfied them.

According to the Bishop of Galway, although the meeting was 'contentious' and he described the Minister as 'truculent', 'the interview ended amicably'. This version of events is consistent with the Minister's report that the Archbishop, 'a courteous host', saw him to the front door – an event witnessed by the Minister's driver.

The Archbishop's version of events, as reported verbally by him to the Taoiseach, is entirely different. He reported that the meeting had been acrimonious and 'incredible' and that the Minister himself had terminated it and walked out.

Regarding the inconsistency in the two Bishops' versions reported above, Noël Browne wrote artfully, 'What a dilemma faces the student of history, deciding which of two bishops was lying about this meeting.'

Believing that his concessions would placate the Bishops, the Minister returned to his Department and prepared a memorandum dealing with all their points. Since 'protocol insisted that a mere Cabinet minister had no direct access to an Archbishop's office', the memorandum was therefore, 'within days' sent to the Taoiseach for immediate forwarding to The Archbishop.

Extraordinarily, the Taoiseach never sent the memorandum to the Bishops. The Minister, assuming that it had been sent, continued with his preparations for the scheme. It languished on the Taoiseach's desk along with the Ferns letter which he had also ignored. Eventually, the final memorandum reached the Hierarchy many months later on 28 March 1951. By this time the Minister's scheme was doomed. During the delay 'Mr Costello was in constant verbal contact with the Archbishop' and the Cabinet took fright. It is extraordinary that Dr Tom O'Higgins, a member of the Cabinet and also a leading light in the IMA, was undoubtedly reporting back the diminishing cabinet support

for the scheme which it had previously endorsed. Noël Browne
reported this conflict of interest damningly in his memoir:

> Fortified by the knowledge that my cabinet colleagues
> had lost their nerve and their enthusiasm for the scheme,
> the consultants became intransigent.

The 'Pamphlet'

While the furtive communication between Taoiseach and
Archbishop continued, and the IMA were encouraged by
faltering cabinet resolve, and the letter from Ferns and the
Minister's reply to it lay festering on the Taoiseach's desk, Noël
Browne pressed on with his preparations. He was masterful
at news management and at the production of populist
documentary materials to promote his scheme. Not least of
these was an explanatory booklet[97] (the Archbishop called it a
pamphlet) which was widely circulated, in which he appealed
to the public, over the heads of the Bishops and the doctors,
and flaunting his democratic mandate and the legitimacy of his
scheme with the irresistible soundbite, 'The people have willed
it'.

Countering the Hierarchy's scaremongering that the scheme
would excessively intrude on the rights of the individual he
states:

> Let me stress the fact that the whole scheme is voluntary.
> Neither, in regard to the mothers and children, will there
> be any compulsion.

This plain talk, completely debunking their phoney
Huxleyite innuendo, can not have pleased Their Lordships.

Then, in a dose of hard facts, the booklet included a bar chart
of infant mortality in most European countries. This graphic
showed Italy, Spain, Belgium and Ireland in a particularly bad
light – all countries in which there was an inverse relationship
between public piety and public health. Having his nose

gratuitously rubbed in such compelling and uncomfortable statistics would have done little for the equanimity of the Archbishop of Dublin. Indeed, it seems fair to say, in view of Spain's starring role, and in deference to its national sport, that the statistics must have been like a red rag to a bull.

The Minister then proceeds to invoke the compatibility of his scheme with the Proclamation of the Republic in 1916 in their mutual objective of 'cherishing all the children of the nation equally'.

This was a particularly apt allusion for a country whose children were dying in numbers far greater than in jurisdictions resorting to more state intervention – precisely that intervention which was being obstructed by the Catholic Hierarchy and the medical establishment.

And then the final flourish. Having belaboured his legitimacy and that of the elected Parliament, he sticks his finger in the Archbishop's eye and throws all his chips on the table with the statement, 'such authority none may refute'.

Sticking a ministerial finger in the eye of the Archbishop of Dublin was no way to get politics done in the Ireland of 1950.

The booklet then proceeds to appeal to the people over the heads of the collective medical profession in terms to which even those of the most marginal Hippocratic persuasion could not reasonably take exception.

> ... all our mothers who choose to avail themselves of the scheme will have at their disposal for themselves and their children all the resources of modern medicine.

> This will be theirs as a right of their nationhood without any mark of the Poor Law, or any means test.

The powerful sentiments expressed here are surely in tune with the teaching of those two, not insignificant, historical figures, Hippocrates and Jesus Christ. The disciples of both however – somewhat astray it would seem – were portraying them as the essence of evil.

Having poked the eye of the Archbishop of Dublin and ignoring the fact that Church and medicine were allied against him, the Minister now goads the doctors with his irresistibly populist declaration that there would be 'no doctors' bills'.

Doctors have always known that they rarely win a slanging match with a politician, who is after votes. It is altogether better to machinate behind the scenes. In 1950, to have the Archbishop of Dublin, John Charles McQuaid, fighting your cause as a proxy was to have achieved the most consummate of machinations. The 'no doctors' bills' proclamation was perceived as a vicious thrust into the purse of medicine. The doyens believed, probably mistakenly, that there would be much leakage of their income through the consequent rent in that purse. This was a time for resort to the back channels of communication between Church and medicine.

With some naïveté the Minister now compounded his already ample difficulties by sending a copy of this booklet to the Archbishop of Dublin – a mistake.

Following receipt of the pamphlet, His Grace, to use an equine metaphor, threw the head. He wrote directly a 'freezing letter'[98] to the Minister for Health on 8 March 1951 in the most peremptory terns, with a copy to the Taoiseach.

> I beg to thank you for your letter of 6th inst. received by me today enclosing a pamphlet which purports to explain the proposed Mother and Child Health Service. I regret however, that, as I stated on the occasion when on behalf of the Hierarchy, I asked you to meet me with Their Lordships of Ferns and Galway, I may not approve the Mother and Child Health Service, as it is proposed by you to implement the Scheme.

This is very much first person singular stuff. 'Their Lordships of Ferns and Galway' are mere adjuncts to the verdict. It is I, John Charles McQuaid, who 'may not approve'.

The letter, though brief, is crafted with cunning. There is no specific mention of the vulgar matter of the means test or the many other vacuous objections which the Hierarchy had raised. Perish the thought that the Archbishop of Dublin should concern himself with such a mundane matter as money. There is, of course, no hint of his concubinage with the doyen doctors. Also there is the devious device of suggesting that it is not so much the scheme itself which is offensive but rather the manner in which 'it is proposed by you to implement' it.

Adroitly, the Archbishop is transferring the odium from the scheme itself to the Minister who is promoting it. Although the letter is addressed to the Minister it is also copied to the Taoiseach and the main signal is intended for the Taoiseach, the head of Government. Paraphrased, the signal to the Taoiseach was intended to be interpreted as follows.

> The problem Dear Taoiseach is not so much with the greater part of the Scheme per se but with your truculent Minister for Health who appears not to understand the established modus vivendi between Church and State. This has the potential greatly to upset that happy equilibrium which is to our mutual benefit. If you can but rid yourself of this turbulent Minister the advantages for both of us will be manifold. For you, Taoiseach, the advantages will be a more tranquil cabinet and by implication a more durable Government. You do not, after all, want to be ejected prematurely by those who have been in power for two decades, who think they own the country, and many of whom have scarcely abandoned the gun. It goes without saying, Taoiseach, that the electoral advantages, in a country so devoutly Catholic and obedient to its Bishops, of the Government being at one with the Hierarchy, are immeasurable.

All of this was, of course, unsaid but conveyed with crystal clarity by those few words, 'I may not approve'.

To be rid of the turbulent Minister, the first to offer them any real show of resistance in the thirty years since the State had been founded, was, of course, a most attractive proposition for the Hierarchy. Noël Browne's approach to things threatened the power of their Caliphate. Because of mankind's tendency to forget even the best lessons of history, the memory of Their Lordships' destruction of Parnell, although lingering, had inevitably faded somewhat over the intervening generations. It was time for a refresher course as to who runs the country. The destruction of this Minister for Health would set the tone for generations to come.

Following the Minister's departure tranquillity would be restored. Ministers would again be respectful and circumspect. Proposed legislation on all sensitive subjects would be submitted to Drumcondra for approval (as de Valera had done with the constitution) well in advance to avoid the potentially catastrophic possibility that 'I may not approve'. For years to come their Lordships would exercise Rasputinesque manipulation of the State, and all of this in a Republic and in secret. Ministers would repair to Drumcondra furtively and, of course, unaccompanied by a civil servant. They would bend the knee and kiss the ring. This latter posture, evocative of the Chinese imperial kowtow, was commonplace at the time and for long after and was expected of all who approached the Episcopal presence.[99] The manoeuvre was extensively and demonstratively practiced by politicians and its vote-catching value more than compensated for any unlikely loss of dignity which the ambitious one might have felt as State bent the knee to Church.

The relevance of all of this to our theme is that, while votes could be garnered in great numbers by deference, knee bending and ring kissing, they could be lost in equal proportion by the merest raising of an Episcopal eyebrow. The doyen doctors, joined with the Bishops in the unholy Episco-Medical alliance, knew all of this. The politicians were the meat in the sandwich. With the exception of the Minister for Health they had, by their servility, lowered themselves to this unenviable status. The doyens of medicine had contrived a situation with only two possible outcomes – the departure of the Minister or the loss of face for the Hierarchy. In the ring kissing Republic of 1950, the latter was never a likely outcome.

POLITICAL BISHOP, SPIRITUAL TAOISEACH

Historians might, of course, offer that there was a third, albeit unlikely, possibility – that the Taoiseach would stand by his Minister and his Republic, politely rebuff Episcopal interference in Government business, and save the country and the Church much future anguish by striking a blow for separation of Church and State. Such a principled stand would, by distancing the Church from the squalor of politics, have greatly fortified the spiritual credibility of the former and the temporal effectiveness of the latter.

Viewed from a distance, however, there was an absurd inversion of the priorities of the respective parties. Their Lordships, for all of their outward spirituality, were more concerned about matters temporal, while the Taoiseach, a man admirable in his unashamed devotion to his religious practices, probably had a more genuine concern for matters spiritual. All of these anxieties, however – the Taoiseach's fear of hell and Drumcondra, Their Lordships fear of losing power and influence and of being consigned to the tedium of spirituality, and the doctors' fear of losing money – converged on one inevitability: the Minister for Health must go.

9

SELF-DESTRUCTING MINISTER

All that remains to be arranged now is the manner of the Minister's departure. It would be altogether more convenient if he could be induced to self-destruct. He must not be allowed to portray himself as a martyr.

Towards the enterprise of inducing him to self-destruct, the Minister himself, by his angularity and rigidity, provided the ideal substrate. While volatile chemistry is rarely prone to spontaneous combustion, the merest spark is often sufficient to set it off. The mercurial Minister was, his integrity notwithstanding – or perhaps, depressingly, because of his over-endowment of that attribute – unsuited to politics. He was in politics in order to achieve certain clearly defined idealistic advances but he lacked the patience to pursue the art of the possible. This enabled his gathering enemies, clerical, medical and political, conveniently to portray him as quixotic. He was now tilting at the very dangerous windmill in Drumcondra and that was the spark that would ignite and consume him – a victim of his own foolishness.

The Taoiseach, the letter from Ferns and the Minister's reply having incubated on his desk for many months like a ticking bomb, finally shook off his torpor and was roused to action. He wrote to the Minister seeking to clarify what was going on between him and the Hierarchy: what had been agreed what was the attitude, as if he did not already know from his many meetings with the Archbishop, of Drumcondra to the Mother and Child Scheme?

Noël Browne wrote back tersely on 19 March 1951:

> Am I correct in thinking that from the terms of your letter of March 15th inst that you are under the impression that the Hierarchy are opposed to the Mother and Child health protection scheme? May I point out that this impression, if held by you, is certainly not borne out by the following facts.

The tone of the Minister's letter is acid; indeed, the vitriol would shortly be flying. While not quite calling his boss a fool, he is less than delicate in suggesting that his assessment is wrong and 'is certainly not borne out by the following facts', facts which, as the letter develops, he lays out with forensic precision. Clearly the Minister for Health and his Taoiseach, at this time, hold diametrically opposing interpretations of what is 'acceptable' to Drumcondra and, more importantly, on the extent to which diktats from that quarter should impact on legislation. It is entirely clear that, while the Minister continues to believe that his scheme is still viable, the Taoiseach has, not to put too fine a point on it, been got at. Government dysfunction has escalated to malfunction.

It was a sign of the times that a Government minister, his unquestionable republican ideology notwithstanding, in his references to the Hierarchy, found it necessary to lapse into an obsequious verbiage more suited to places governed by emperors, oligarchs, ayatollahs and their unelected elites. The title Archbishop of Dublin had every time to be prefixed by 'His Grace'. Neither would the functional monikers Bishop of Galway or Bishop of Ferns suffice in reference to those clerical gentlemen who became 'Their Lordships'. Some may argue that the use of such titles was no more than good manners. It is hard to escape the conclusion, however, that the lines were unevenly drawn when the untitled representatives of the State did business with such grandeur.

The Minister might at this time have been well advised to organise an orderly retreat in order to fight another day. Catastrophically, he appears to have been unaware of or ignored the fact that the Cabinet were wilting before the Episcopal onslaught. His party leader in particular, Sean McBride, notwithstanding his history of violent republicanism, was caving in to the Bishops. Failing, however, to appreciate his tactical dilemma, and confused by the conflict between idealism and *realpolitik*, he persisted in his grand strategy in pursuit of which he continued to throw himself upon the ramparts of Drumcondra where he must surely perish as had so many before.

Referring to his infamous meeting with the three Bishops at Drumcondra, the Minister berates the Taoiseach:

> I gave you to understand I was quite satisfied in my mind that the misapprehensions which were referred to by His Grace and their Lordships at that meeting were satisfactorily disposed of.

There is an air of unreality about this statement which undermines somewhat the Minister's credibility. It is March 1951. The Bishops are up in arms as never before; the Cabinet is destabilised and showing signs of disintegrating and he is beleaguered on all sides. Instead of taking stock of his position he resorts to indignation – a poor substitute for *realpolitik*.

The Minister then concedes that while he had reached agreement with the Bishops on all other issues there was 'one outstanding point concerning health education.'

The Minister refers, almost *en passant*, to this one outstanding point. Everything else, according to him, apart from this one residual detail, was settled with the Bishops. The 'one outstanding point', however, was code for the possibility that, in the eyes of the Bishops, the scheme might lead to the introduction of contraception and in due course other associated evils in the reproductive domain. Alas for the Minister it related to the Catholic Church's enduring and disproportionate obsession with all things sexual and reproductive. In the view of Their Lordships the Minister's proposal for 'health education' raised the appalling prospect of reproduction being transformed from a lottery to a science.

The national reproduction lottery in 1950 held the nation in its grip. The lottery was, above all others, the device by which Their Lordships kept the nation, and particularly its women, in thrall. The hippopotamus in the parlour at Drumcondra, therefore, was the appalling spectre that the exceedingly fecund Catholic women of Ireland might be educated and equipped with the knowledge and apparatus to control their legendary reproductive profligacy. That much honoured matriarch of the labour ward, the Grand Multipara[100] – defined for medical students of the time as a woman who produced ten or more foot-soldiers for the Church militant – would be no more.

Indeed, so Their Lordships' reasoning went, had not the Protestants of Ireland, greatly to the detriment of their numbers, long since abandoned the reproductive lottery using methods and devices devised by the devil himself, and which would surely condemn them to join their inventor in the everlasting flames of hell.

The Hierarchy, however, considered and taught that members of other Churches and creeds were beyond salvation: their Faustian pact was of no interest to them. His Grace would spare his own flock from the devil's implements which interfered with reproduction. Pregnancy, or its avoidance, would remain a lottery predictable with no more certainty, or perhaps less, than the result of the three-fifteen at Punchestown. For Catholics running in the reproduction stakes Their Lordships would ensure that the going remained heavy. His Grace would sell his regime in the manner of a strapped Minister for Finance presenting a hairshirt budget – pain today, jam tomorrow.

The Catholic Hierarchy's view, in 1950, of what constituted 'health education' was extraordinary. The country was unwashed and malnourished.[101] Dentition was diabolical. Diphtheria, whooping cough, meningitis, tuberculosis, gastroenteritis and a host of other miseries were rife and dreaded by the people. The diseases of dirt and deprivation were everywhere. Worse still were the diseases of ignorance. Nutritional diseases were commonplace. Centuries after the Royal Navy, by education, eliminated scurvy, this entirely avoidable disease was still found in Irish children and was to be seen in the hospital wards of this writer's medical education many years later. Rickets shamefully, as discussed earlier, in a country awash with milk, was likewise seen in the wards, featured in clinical examinations, and continued to ravage the skeletons of children well into the 1960s and beyond.

This surely is the stuff with which 'health education' should have been concerning itself.

The Minister then proceeds, in the most unequivocal terms, to say that he had reassured the Bishops that his scheme would not introduce anything which ran counter to Catholic moral teaching.

> I gave unequivocal guarantees to His Grace and their Lordships that everything possible which could be done to allay their fears in this regard I would most willingly carry out, if necessary in forthcoming amending legislation to the 1947 Health Act.

It is clear that the Minister was willing to accommodate the Bishops with regard to any moral reservations they might have about his scheme. He is, in effect, calling their bluff. On such a doctrinaire Catholic matter as contraception in 1950 they felt certain that the people would follow their advice blindly: the Bishops say the scheme is morally repugnant – that is enough for us. The people, however, were not to be told that the Minister was prepared to accommodate the Bishop's wishes entirely in this regard. When the Minister declared himself willing to change the law if necessary to accommodate the Bishop's 'fears', the moral dimension should have been completely removed but with it would go Their Lordship's leverage on the population.

If, on the other hand the Bishops overtly declared themselves against the scheme because it was completely free, the moral leverage would be lost and their message would be a much more difficult sell. Even their erudite Lordships could not argue a connection between a means test and the everlasting flames of hell. The Archbishop of Dublin had painted himself into a corner and the only way he could extricate himself was by insisting on the phoney moral dimension.

The Minister had sent his explanatory 'pamphlet' not only to McQuaid but to all the Bishops and a number acknowledged receipt.

> In none of these acknowledgements is there any suggestion of any objection to the Scheme, except in the letter from His Grace the Archbishop of Dublin.

Again in this passage the Minister's naïveté and failure to grasp the rudiments of *realpolitik* are exposed. He has generated explanatory literature regarding his scheme and has circulated it. That he should feel obliged to circulate a proposal for the advancement of healthcare to each and every member of the Hierarchy, rather than to the cognate disciplines in medicine, demonstrates the extent to which Church and State had merged with the latter subsumed by the former to the detriment of both.

Acknowledgement of correspondence is no more than common civility and the Minister was naïve in interpreting such acknowledgement as acquiescence. Such Bishops as approved of the scheme – and there were undoubtedly some who saw nothing wrong with it – knew better than to reply in writing to the Archbishop's enemy, the Minister, saying, 'good man, carry on'. Also there were many Bishops from rural dioceses who did not amount to what Noël Browne scathed as 'political Bishops' and these would have been completely dominated by the metropolitan McQuaid and his kitchen cabinet of 'Ferns' and 'Galway'. These latter rural Bishops, and any who thought like them, confined themselves to polite acknowledgement, misinterpreted by the Minister as acquiescence, and were happy to keep the head down and allow the main man in Drumcondra to make the running.

There is a transient flash of worldliness and insight in the Minister's gambit of laying the blame squarely on the Archbishop while exculpating many of his Episcopal colleagues. The beneficiary of an Anglo-Saxon education, he is acquainted with perfidious Albion's well-tried device of 'divide and rule', and he now seeks to separate, in the Taoiseach's mind, the generality of Their Lordships from their commander in chief in Drumcondra.

Noël Browne points out to the Taoiseach that he has in fact been in touch with a member of the Hierarchy who has told him that:

> ... so far as he is aware, the Hierarchy as such have expressed no objection to the Mother and Child Scheme whatsoever on the grounds of faith and morals.

The matter of 'faith and morals' is important, if a little tedious, to consider.

It should be remembered that Noël Browne is still, at this time, a convinced Catholic. He has genuinely sincere concerns about the issue of 'faith and morals' and he wants to be sure, since he is jousting with the Church's top brass, of his theological ground. In order to satisfy his conscience he displays the same methodical approach as in the earlier matter of his deficiency in the Irish language – he consults a distinguished theologian for help and advice. He takes that step, as does a wise clinical doctor in a difficult situation in practice, of seeking outside opinion before the need to do so is forced upon him.

This consultation, he reveals in his memoir, takes place at length and in secret. That the consultation should have to take place in secret, not least for the protection of he who was consulted, was indicative of the menace with which the disciple of Machiavelli in Drumcondra ruled. The distinguished Professor of Moral Theology at Maynooth seminary, who advised the Minister, was not outed[102] for many years and was thus spared the fate of a colleague in that institution who bravely spoke out against scandalous abuses and was rusticated to obscurity in the West.[103]

The theologian drew a clear distinction between matters of faith and morals which were absolute, and Church teaching which was arbitrary. He advised that, in his opinion, with regard to faith and morals there could be no impediment whatever to the Minister's scheme. Indeed, a less erudite observer than the said professor might be tempted to suggest that it was not the Minister's scheme which was an affront to faith and morals but rather the Archbishop's resistance to it.

Then Noël Browne, with the desperation of the damned, throws all caution to the winds by demanding of the hapless Taoiseach:

> ... whether your withholding of approval to the Mother and Child Scheme is due either to the supposed opposition of the Hierarchy to the Scheme or to the possible opposition of any individual member of the Hierarchy.

The Minister is doing that which does not always go down well in politics: he is calling a spade a spade – almost. The spade in this case is the Archbishop of Dublin. The Minister, however, displaying uncharacteristic circumspection, even now feels unable to go as far as actually naming the villain. He seeks instead, with very considerable naïveté, to induce the

Taoiseach into naming the Archbishop. In doing so he shows poor comprehension of Costello's predicament or insight into his character.

Notwithstanding that Noël Browne had tooled himself up theologically, and although merely a medical doctor, he now felt that he could debate the issue on equal terms with the Drumcondra Doctor of Divinity. There would be no such debate. The great autocrat, falling back upon the power of his office, the passivity of the people and the politicians, did not do debate. Shakespeare got it again: 'I am Sir Oracle, and when I ope my lips let no dog bark.'[104]

10

THE EPISCOPAL BRIEF

Then as now the legislature was well, perhaps excessively, endowed with lawyers. The Taoiseach was by trade a barrister and by all accounts loved practicing at the Bar. He was thus a member of that sect deeply embedded in the establishment. He brought to the office of Taoiseach three attributes which made him extremely unlikely to wish to puncture the Episcopal hegemony to which Ireland was captive.

Firstly, the Taoiseach, John A. Costello had been recognised as an able practitioner at the Bar. In order to practice at that profession it is necessary to have a well-developed sense of credulity – one must manage to believe in the justice of the client's cause regardless how lost it might seem in the eyes of lesser mortals. It is of course axiomatic that everybody is entitled to a defence and this pseudo-belief in the rectitude of even the most villainous, enables the barrister to mount a defence with the greatest purity and conviction. Apparently during his days at the Bar the incumbent Taoiseach had, even by the standards of his own credulous profession, excelled at this device of self-deception. On accepting a brief he could, regardless of its merits, argue the case with commendable conviction – a great man to have in one's corner. A man who could so readily slip into convinced mode at the briefing of mere legal colleagues was likely quickly to succumb to the persuasions of one so great as the Archbishop of Dublin. He embraced the Episcopal brief, its dubious merits notwithstanding, with his accustomed ease and conviction.

The brief however was like no other that the barrister Taoiseach had ever received: it did not arrive on his desk in documentary form but rather by way of informal communication and innuendo. It differed also in one other profound respect as follows. When a barrister receives his brief and does his stuff he usually gets paid regardless of the result, win lose or draw – nice work if you can get it. This Episcopal brief however came with no such comforts. The consequences of failure, which in this instance meant failure to destroy the Minister and his scheme, would be dire for the barrister Taoiseach. Not only would he receive no award of costs but the Taxing Master of Drumcondra would dish out punitive damages in the form of a shower of pious vitriol calculated to unsettle the electorate, unseat the fractious coalition government and consign it, the Taoiseach, his turbulent Minister and his unholy scheme to oblivion.

Such was the unappetising fate which, in the unhappy event of his failing to do things the easy way, awaited the hapless Taoiseach. Hapless he was because it was particularly ironic for a Taoiseach who, during a recent trip abroad and with much fanfare, had impromptu officially announced that Ireland would abandon its *demi-monde* status of 'Free State' and henceforth posture as a Republic.[105] Now alas he would be remembered for submitting, in a most un-republican way, to the diktats of unelected sectional religious interests.

THE CROZIER OF DAMOCLES

The sword of Damocles, from its mythical and metaphoric origins, had taken on various physical forms throughout history: its manifestation in Ireland in 1950 was the crozier. This implement, from its humble pastoral origins, had developed into an impressive accessory worthy of its bearers. The presence of the crozier, rather like that of the mace sported by many great institutions on formal occasions, symbolised power. The crozier, sparingly exhibited today, was ubiquitous in 1950. Their Lordships, if we might borrow a phrase, never left home without it.

The crozier, while serving as an added decoration to their already much gilded Lordships, and while lacking the military origins and symbolism of the mace, did nevertheless have utilitarian function – as an instrument of political chastisement in Ireland it had no equal. When swung in chastising mode – and there was ample precedent for this manoeuvre in Ireland – anybody caught within its metaphoric radius ended up severely bruised.

The Archbishop of Dublin had a crozier the radius of which when swung was, as one might expect, in direct proportion to the power of his office. The area of the circle thus described was very great indeed. The incumbent Taoiseach knew that he was well within the ambit of the swinging crozier. This sobering realisation, coupled with his barrister's flexibility of mind, enabled him comfortably to accommodate to the Archbishop's point of view. Indeed, it is likely that he slipped with ease into the convenient belief that the national interest would now be best served by ridding himself of this albatross of a Minister.

LAME DUCK TAOISEACH

The second factor which made the Taoiseach unlikely to resist Church bullying was his own lack of credibility. It was a unique circumstance that Costello was not, at the time of the election which brought his party to power, leader of that party. The actual leader was Richard Mulcahy, a man of iron will who, in order to prevent anarchy, had during a bitter civil war in the new State ordered the reprisal execution of prisoners in highly dubious circumstances. Mulcahy as leader found himself, in his attempts to assemble a patchwork coalition, dependent upon the support of associates of the executed ones and they detested him. He was also politically more savvy than Costello and would have been less malleable in the hands of Bishops. The party leader, however, with 'remarkable selflessness'[106] stepped aside to be replaced, as Taoiseach, by his more acceptable and altogether more ductile party colleague. It has been suggested that John A. Costello, whose primary interest had always been practising at the Bar, accepted the great office of Taoiseach with reluctance.[107]

The Taoiseach therefore came to office as something of a political lame duck – not at all the one to lead such an experimental and bockety coalition. The lame duck was a poor match for the sure-footed senior prelate of the Church rampant and the doyens of medicine knew it. The medical cognoscenti calculated, correctly, that a man of the Taoiseach's background, temperament and vulnerability would – notwithstanding the absurdity of the issue – buckle every time when confronted with the might of Drumcondra.

And the absurdity of the issue should be reiterated. It was simply whether a much needed medical regime, agreed by all but the higher echelons of medicine to be desirable, should or should not be means tested.

An added complication for the Taoiseach was that his family was connected, at first degree relative level, to the family of certain of the dons and doyens of medicine. The Archbishop was chairman of the board of the don's hospital and there was more than ample opportunity to pour medical propaganda into the ear of His Grace. The furtive proceedings of such encounters could then be passed through the family conduit back to the Taoiseach. All of this must have had a salutary effect on the unfortunate head of Government walking a tightrope between the Archbishop's palace and restive leftish elements of his cabinet.

HOLY WRIT

The third factor which made the Taoiseach unlikely to flout the Bishops was his Catholic orthodoxy. In all that he said and did he honourably conceded his loyalty to his Church. To him, what the Bishops said was holy writ.

11

EDUCATION AND SCIENTIFIC ADVANCE

The Minister for Health was of the view that the people of Ireland, and not least the women, were in need of education with regard to healthcare and he was preparing to legislate accordingly. The relevant Section 21 of the Act, with admirable brevity read:

> A health authority shall, in accordance with regulations made under section 28 of this Act make arrangements for safeguarding the health of women in respect of motherhood and *for their education in that respect* (Italics added).

It was to this latter clause (in italics) that John Charles McQuaid took extreme exception and it is clear from what follows, that this had been discussed between the Archbishop and the Taoiseach.

The Taoiseach, whom we have accused of earlier ignoring the issue in the hope that it would go away, now realises that it will consume him and his Government if he does not act. He had in fact written to the Minister days earlier (15 March, 1951) regurgitating all the objections set out in 'Ferns' letter of October 1950. In this letter the Taoiseach betrays his supine mentality by accusing his Minister of the heinous crime of 'defiance of the Hierarchy'.

Roused to fury by his Minister's unyielding and impertinent reply, the Taoiseach's response is immediate on 21 March 1951, and is increasingly sulphurous. Much of the letter is a pathetic further recitation of the Hierarchy's objection to the Scheme. In reading the correspondence one is tempted to the view that the Taoiseach had no original thoughts or arguments of his own. His position was that the Scheme must die simply because the Hierarchy were against it.

> My withholding of approval of the scheme is due to the objections set forth in the letter to me from the Secretary to the Hierarchy, and to the reiteration of their objections by his Grace the Archbishop of Dublin, as Archbishop of Dublin.

The Taoiseach was thus prepared to concede to the Archbishop of Dublin a veto on proposed legislation and is unashamedly writing that his Minister for Health must comply with that veto. It is clear that the Taoiseach had no idea whatsoever, his legal training notwithstanding, of what might be an appropriate relationship between Church and State in a Republic – the very Republic which he, with fanfare and more than a little petulance, had declared himself in the recent past. He did, however, try his hand at a little matchmaking by offering as follows:

> ... my personal help to you as intermediary with the Hierarchy to try to smooth those difficulties and resolve their objections which I felt could be done by appropriate amendments of the scheme and amending legislation if necessary.

The Taoiseach then goes on to suggest to his Minister how the Health Act, 1947 might be amended in order to accommodate the Bishops' objections. If the Minister could see his way to delete the clause on the education of women it might yet be possible to meet the objections of the Bishops.

THE DANGERS OF EDUCATION

The word 'education', as used here, means of course the appalling prospect that doctors might disclose to women biological secrets about the functioning of their own reproductive apparatus. The Taoiseach was offering his 'intermediary' services as midwife to bring into the world a Health Act free from this educational taint.

The Archbishop, in exhibiting this fear of 'education', will be derided by many as stupid: the opposite however is the case – he was showing himself to be calculating and prescient.

There were two main pillars supporting the Catholic Church's breeding policy for its flock.

The first was male domination. It is hardly surprising that the Church should promote its own patriarchal model amongst lay society. Although the clergy were themselves, for the most part, celibate, they nevertheless, since it suited their purpose, displayed a sympathetic understanding of the biological urges and requirements of the male of the species. They were, therefore, big on the rather quaintly named issue of 'conjugal rights'. It was, according to Church teaching, the prerogative of the male to exercise these 'rights' according to his immediate urge and, in a country where the main plank of the economy was the production, marketing and consumption of porter and a plethora of other alcoholic beverages, this boded ill for restraint and well for the continuation of the reproduction lottery and for the recruitment of foot soldiers into the Church militant.

Was the female of the species after all not referred to in the Bible as the vessel,[108] a mere carrying apparatus which after nine months discharged itself and was intended by nature to be immediately replenished? Whether the women of 1950 carried their status of 'vessel' philosophically or with resignation, and the latter seems distinctly more likely, there was little prospect of emancipation while Their Lordships of the Hierarchy held sway – a situation which would prevail well into the future.

Their Lordships therefore felt entirely secure with regard to the first pillar of their power, male domination. They continued to require that the concept of (female) obedience be enshrined in the text of the marriage vows, and this was accepted by a docile population without demur. This was, after all, an indigenous Irish cultural matter best determined by those who took upon themselves the moral stewardship of the nation.

The second pillar upon which the Bishops' breeding policy for the nation balanced in 1950 was women's fertility and their complete lack of control over it. This pillar was secure enough but by no means taken for granted by the prescient one in Drumcondra. The women of Ireland, at that time as distinct from later, tended to marry young and were thus in peak reproductive fettle. The production line was secure so long as there was no resort to diabolical methods and accoutrements which might enable women artificially to control that fertility. The Minister for Health was proposing 'education' for women in these matters – in the eyes of the Hierarchy an appalling vista.

THE UNIVERSITY OF CHICAGO AND KING CANUTE

The doyens of medicine, including certain professors of obstetrics and gynaecology, were of course well up to speed with the galloping pace of scientific developments in the reproductive arena. These medical gentlemen would have been pouring into the receptive ear of His Grace tidings of a most alarming kind.

The Archbishop would doubtless have been appraised of the burgeoning research in steroid chemistry then afoot in the United States. By 1950, synthesised female sex hormones were beginning to emerge from laboratories at the University of Chicago[109] and elsewhere. These compounds, showing every promise of being amenable to mass production, could theoretically be used to regulate the female reproductive cycle. The intense interest in these developments displayed by powerful pharmaceutical companies, who were throwing money at the research, was proof positive that they foresaw a lucrative mass market. They were intent, the Archbishop would have been told, on producing – horror of horrors – a pill which quite simply could prevent women getting pregnant.

The mass production of pills – the story went – would put an end to the mass production of babies. The reproductive lottery would be no more; the three-fifteen at Punchestown would always be won by the favourite and, in a boringly predictable world, the ace in Their Lordships pack, the Grand Multipara, would be consigned to history. And all the while the doyens of obstetrics and gynaecology were doing no more than discharging their convenient moral duty to inform His Grace of the impending threat to this fundamental pillar of his power.

There is an attractive concept in medicine of the translation of the fruits of research from laboratory to patient – from bench to bed so to speak. In the topic under discussion, however, the Godless research would, in the view of the Hierarchy, translate not to the hospital, but to the conjugal bed. Events in the conjugal bed at this time were very much the business of their celibate Lordships. It was, of course, difficult in 1950 to predict how long it would take for events in the University of Chicago to invade the conjugal bed in Ireland, but there was a certain scientific inevitability that the project would succeed. Their Lordships therefore adhered to the wise axiom, then taught to every child in Ireland, that prevention is better than cure. The Hierarchy therefore swung into double prevention mode: they would prevent the prevention of pregnancy.

It is without doubt that the Irish Church was doing no more than adhering to the Canute policy emanating from Rome. It is, however, hard to escape the conclusion that they were applying that policy with a vigour which their peers in other countries did not find necessary. In most other countries Church and State had long since separated in an enlightened mutual respect. In Ireland the mutuality was lopsided and Their Lordships, being in the ascendant, were not yet ready for such a divorce.

In the event, if we might digress briefly in a fast forward direction, the prognostications of the doyens of medicine, and the prescient forebodings of the Archbishop, were vindicated. What had seemed unthinkable in 1950 came to pass ten years later when, in 1960, the United States Food and Drug Administration licensed for general use the dreaded pill.[110] Their Lordships, with their supine politicians of all hues in tow, then launched into Canute overdrive, and indeed with considerable success. Manipulating the State, for a time they held back the march of science but were all the while advancing into a quixotic cul de sac. Even John Charles McQuaid could not succeed where Canute had failed.

We have conceded that His Grace of Drumcondra showed himself to be prescient in these matters. This view is supported by the writings of none less than the German Nobel Laureate and *habitué* of the west of Ireland, Heinrich Boll. Boll, disillusioned with his own country, decamped to the west of Ireland where, around this time, he wrote his *Irish Journal* published in 1957.[111] A Catholic himself, he described with affection the culture, ambience, simplicity and large families to be found in his Western European Atlantic idyll in Achill Island. Returning to Ireland years later he found, to his regret, the country profoundly transformed, and the main agent of this transformation he described as 'His majesty the pill'.

But in 1950 all of this was still in the future. The Archbishop had allowed himself to be manoeuvred into a somewhat Talibanesque position where he was resisting 'education' for women. The absurdity of this position would have discomforted lesser mortals but not John Charles McQuaid. Egged on by the doyens of medicine he sticks to his guns and war breaks out everywhere. The Hierarchy, a formidable foe, is at war with the Minister for Health. The Minister is at war with his Taoiseach. The Minister is also at war with his party leader Sean McBride, a man with whom it was not difficult to disagree. The Minister was at open war with the doctors, the exchanges rising to a level of bellicosity far in excess of the default relationship between medicine and Government in Ireland which is that of a frozen conflict. And worst of all, if the Taoiseach does not bend the knee, a major conflict is in the offing between Church and State.

During all of this the people were, of course, aware that there was tension between the medical leadership and the Minister for Health. For the public this must have been confusing. This was, after all, the Minister who had done so much for them. Hospitals had been built, tuberculosis had been tackled and showed signs of yielding, and now a scheme was proposed which would, free of charge, improve the comfort and safety of childbearing women. The scheme would furthermore, again free of charge, support the health and nutrition of all children up to the age of sixteen years.

It was not, however, the opposition of the medical establishment to the scheme which confused the public. Such opposition was perceived as nothing more noble than the protection of vested interest and would have been unsurprising to most. Doctors then, as now, were considered by the citizens to possess more than their fair share of whatever money was around. It is true that, in a more simple time, the vulgar abusive moniker of 'fat cat' – so beloved of the left – did not enjoy such currency as it does today. Nevertheless, the people, then and since, were happy to surrender themselves easily to the comfort of doublethink. They looked with trust and indeed affection upon their own doctor. They did not however lavish this affection on the organised medical profession generally, and especially when it was, as now, in negotiating mode.

The Minister was, after all, sitting on the barrel, doling out pork[112] to his supporters – a largesse which was unlikely to confuse or alienate them. The people were, however, confused by persistent reports that the Church was against the Mother and Child Scheme.

12

A Bad Time to Pick a Fight

In order to appreciate the unequal contest in which the Minister now found himself, it is opportune to reflect on the religious fervour which gripped Ireland in 1950. The word fervour is not here used pejoratively, but rather to emphasise the disastrous judgement and lack of subtlety of the Minister in trying to swim, as he put it in his memoir, 'against the tide'.

The year 1950 had been declared by the Vatican, then usually referred to as the Holy See, a Holy Year. The Papal Bull,[113] harbinging this religious extravaganza, was greeted in Ireland with the greatest possible enthusiasm. A plethora of pious projects and devotional events was arranged and trumpeted in the news media. The country hung on every word of *L'Osservatore Romano*[114] as interpreted for the citizens by the national broadcaster. Much that was good came out of this enthusiasm. It was not, however, a propitious environment in which for the Minister for Health to find himself in a fight with the Church of Rome.

Structural evidence still remains of the religious enthusiasm which gripped the country at precisely the time when the Minister for Health foolishly jousted with the Bishops. Amongst the most conspicuous symbols, still adorning the countryside from that time, are the mountaintop crosses. These monumental structures represented the best in community spirit and voluntary effort. While they have remained more sturdy than the faith that created them, they have further imprinted Christianity on a landscape already much decorated by more venerable and ancient structures. They mock political correctness and have become part of the heritage.[115] Such crosses have become the venue for local community events and celebrations as well as touristic visits. Many an otherwise unpretentious parish is proud, in a more secular age, to sustain such a monument.

The rediscovery and dusting off of ancient Mass rocks, ubiquitous throughout the country and dating from the time of persecution of the majority religion, became commonplace. Again, many of these informal heritage sites are maintained by commendable local community effort and are of immense interest to our returning diaspora.

That which most epitomised the religious zeal of the time, however, has left no mark on the landscape.

The parish mission was the set *pièce de resistance* of the time and, not surprisingly, these increased dramatically in frequency and intensity. The mission achieved its most florid expression in rural Ireland. The format was well worked out. Journeymen 'missioners', usually in the form of Redemptorists working in pairs, arrived and stayed a week. The mode of communication was by fulmination. The mission of these journeymen was decidedly biased towards the negative – hell got much more air-time than heaven. They dispensed much fire and brimstone. They were, above all, masters of the dramatic. The drama gathered to a crescendo on closing night. In darkened Church, with lighted candles held aloft, the devil was renounced 'with all his works and pomps' and even the most recidivist wretches vowed, having unburdened themselves, to sin no more.

Such was the febrile atmosphere in which the Minister for Health, Dr Noël Browne, was increasingly seen to be in disagreement with the Bishops.

INDULGENCES

According to the Papal Bull, 1950 was to be a year of pilgrimage – to Rome. This was a very practical, indeed one might even say a worldly, proposition. A trip to Rome, in the Ireland of 1950, was a very great extravagance indeed. Furthermore, those who could afford to travel were drawn disproportionately from the three groups we are discussing – religious, political and medical. The Pope, however, in order to soften the blow, resorted to an old ploy – the granting of indulgences. Those who could afford to undertake the journey would be the beneficiaries of plenary indulgences.[116] The sinful slate of Dives would thus be wiped clean. Meanwhile, poor old Lazarus, unable to afford such a quick fix for his transgressions, would, as usual, have to take his chances at home. Little in fact had changed since the year 1520 when Martin Luther, exasperated by the abuse and commercialisation of indulgences, was driven out by another Papal Bull.[117]

While Luther had nailed his principles to the Church door at Wittenberg, the Government of the Irish Church–State complex nailed its colours to the Papal mast. They decided to decamp *en masse*, in the manner of the Islamic Haj, to Rome in pursuit of indulgences. It was indeed considered at the time that this junketing – for such is what we would now call it – reflected great credit on the Irish nation and enabled its politicians and prelates to represent themselves to His Holiness the Pope as arch enemies of his *bête noir*, communism.

The Minister for Health, Dr Noël Browne, however, had not gone to Rome. He decided, adhering to the much touted maxim of the time, *laborare est orare*,[118] that, forsaking indulgences, he would stay at home along with Lazarus and attend to the running of his department in the hope of improving the wretched lot of the latter. In the febrile religiosity of the time this impious delinquency did not go unnoticed and afforded McCarthyite elements the opportunity to stigmatise his efforts to produce good public health services as communist.

STAMPS AND STATUES

The intense Catholic ethos permeated all areas of the Church–State. In a time of limited travel opportunity – the indulgence-hunting junketeers being a conspicuous exception – postage stamps afforded an insight into the essence of many countries. Amid the religious enthusiasm of the Holy Year it was felt that Ireland should display its piety through its postal service with a special commemorative stamp, thus reassuring its diaspora and others that, in spite of the perilous state of the world generally, all was well in the Island of Saints and Scholars.

Material of the greatest ecclesiastical, historical and archaeological importance was available in abundance to showcase the treasures of the nation – an opportunity not to be missed.

It was not, however, any ancient ecclesiastical site or edifice which was depicted on the stamps. Many such ancient and venerable sites associated with the Saints and Scholars were, of course, available for display but they did not fit the agenda.

The agenda was to demonstrate that the Irish State was inextricably bound to Rome. It is likely that the State sought Episcopal advice as to what might be suitable subject material for the commemorative stamps. In any case, what appeared on the stamps was not Clonmacnoise, Skeilig Micil or the Rock of Cashel. Indeed, the Book of Kells would have provided the most excellent subject material but alas, like the unfortunate Minister for Health, the odds were stacked against it. Both the Minister and the great illuminated manuscript shared the curse of being associated with Trinity College, an educational establishment in which their Catholic Lordships had 'no confidence'. The opportunity, therefore, to showcase the great ecclesiastical treasures of the nation, with the dual benefit of honouring the Holy Year and promoting tourism, was spurned.

What appeared on the strikingly austere and anticlimactic stamps was an obscure statue of St Peter, which was housed in his eponymous basilica in Rome. It can be assumed with some confidence that the mandarins of the Department of Posts and Telegraphs and their Minister[119] would have been less than familiar with this artefact. Clearly, the daft choice was made by the Hierarchy and probably by Dr McQuaid who was a *habitué* of the Eternal City. The crass absurdity of this was apparent to none. Few questioned why it was that the Irish Postal Service saw fit to act as a recruiting agent for the Italian tourist industry.

The said industry had little need of this support. In his prescription for indulgences the Pope had made it clear that travellers to Rome could, without impairing their kudos with the almighty and thus forfeiting their indulgences, take the opportunity to travel more widely and savour the classical, climatic and oenological delights of Italy generally. Thus began, from this humble beginning – and bearing in mind the axiom that all beginnings are small – the great modern phenomenon of the Irish politician travelling in style and at public expense to exotic locations to represent the taxpayer who could not himself aspire to such grandeur. The delinquency of Noël Browne, in not travelling to Rome with the rest of the Cabinet, would not have escaped the attention of His Grace in Drumcondra.

BROADCASTING SPECTACULAR

The national broadcaster long before television but ever populist, was happy to join in the orgy of religiosity. In his conflict with the Bishops, over the development of the Health Service, the Minister could expect little dissenting support or discordant analysis to come over the airwaves. Broadcasting policy, like political policy, was sanitised by passage through the filter of Drumcondra.

The broadcasting denizens of the GPO – for it is there that they resided in simpler times – decided to do a 'spectacular'. There would be, for the first time, a live outside broadcast from

Europe. This was a daunting technological challenge for the time, but the rewards of bringing the Holy Year opening extravaganza live to the Irish faithful would more than compensate for the effort, expense and inconvenience. The inconvenience would, as in the case of the pilgrims and politicians, involve arduous travel to Italy for a sizeable party on behalf of the taxpayer. It is not possible, at this remove, to know if this broadcast could have been achieved more economically. Could, for example, the much touted *Osservatore Romano* have hot-wired its stuff to Dublin for local interpretation into the vernacular? Better still, could Vatican Radio, possessed of the hardware and skills, have been pressed into service? But none of these would have been the real McCoy and the proper example was, in any case, being set by the junketing politicians

The denizens of the GPO, therefore, like the earlier revolutionary occupants of that historic place, would not be found wanting. The dignity of the occasion, and the pious nation that they represented, demanded travel and travel they must. And so it came to pass that the flower of Irish broadcasting, mindful that indulgences could not be transmitted by wire, decamped lock, stock and barrel, bell, book, candle and microphone, for the Eternal City to report the great happening live to a waiting nation.

The broadcasters did something else which, to their credit, was entirely original, popular, inexpensive, involved neither indulgences nor junketing and has endured over the intervening six decades into the digital age. They decided to broadcast the Angelus. It is likely that this was done at the behest of the Archbishop of Dublin who had an interest in horology and was a stickler for precision and punctuality. It was engineered that at noon and 6.00 pm precisely, the automated peals of the Pro-Cathedral would ring out their call to prayer to be wired simultaneously to the GPO, and thence transmitted to the entire nation in temporal juxtaposition to major news bulletins.

Indeed, such news bulletins in 1950 increasingly featured the gathering controversy over the Mother and Child scheme and the conflict between the renegade Minister for Health and the doyens of medicine and Church.

It seems unlikely that the Archbishop of Dublin was an admirer of the Islamic faith. He was, however, entirely ready to resort to Islamic methods in the form of punctuated public calls to prayer. And much better than the labour-intensive method of the Muezzin repeatedly climbing to his minaret to give forth was the automatic and totally reliable transmission of the peals of the Pro-Cathedral bell into every home in the land – one of His Grace's rare concessions to modernity.

These observations should not in the least be interpreted as censorious of the broadcasting of the Angelus. Rather, in modern more secular times, the bell serves the therapeutic purpose of affording a moment of tranquillity, reflection and exhalation in a more driven world. The story, however, serves to remind those who would forget, or deny, the extent to which one man held the country, its institutions including its publicly funded medical institutions and its body politic in his grip.

And so the Angelus rang out across the country in 1950, but alas, the hapless Minister for Health, Dr Noël Browne, was the one for whom the bell tolled.

PRIMARY EDUCATION

It is axiomatic that indoctrination, if it is to be effective, is best begun early – 'the child is father of the man'.[120] The religious fervour which swept the country came out of the primary schools. It produced cradle Catholics. It finds its modern parallel in the madrassas of Pakistan and elsewhere. The teachers were as active in promoting Catholic orthodoxy as were the clergy – on occasion more so. A vignette from the author's childhood experience will serve to exemplify this.

The year was 1952 and the power and prestige of the Church, along with that of John Charles McQuaid, were at their zenith.

The country was to be honoured by a most auspicious visitation. Francis Cardinal Spellman, Cardinal Archbishop of New York and jewel in the crown of the American Catholic Irish diaspora, was to visit the land of his ancestors.[121] Halleluiah.

The visit of a foreign prelate was always a *cause célèbre* and the national airwaves were saturated with his every peregrination and utterance. In the little country schoolhouse of two teachers, where religious instruction often trumped the three Rs, there was much discussion and anticipation of the great man's visit to Ireland. The ocean liner not yet having yielded to the aircraft, the great man would arrive in splendour at the transatlantic port of Cobh – possibly the same from which his antecedents had departed in markedly contrasting squalor. Thence he would be whisked, by a special Great Southern Railways train, coal not yet having yielded to diesel, to the nation's capital. The trains, ever a source of fascination for the children, ran and rattled hard by the little schoolhouse. The headmaster, ultra Catholic and an austere enforcer of the Archbishop's dreary regime, decided that the passage of the celebrity prelate through his patch must be marked by a display of loyal enthusiasm and obeisance.

The itinerary of Spellman was avidly charted, and on the appointed day all the children were lined up at the station in the manner of a guard of honour to wave the great man through. The event was evanescent. The train belched through at terrifying speed and proximity, the great one oblivious of and indeed well accustomed to the homage. The event may have been transitory, indeed the little station has also yielded, but the memory was embedded to be disinterred later in a wiser world.

It emerged in due course[122] that the said Cardinal Archbishop, notwithstanding his acknowledged ability, was a sexually promiscuous and licentious practitioner of much that he and his Church overtly condemned and victimised. This writer rankles at having been used, as was the schoolmaster in good faith, to honour him.

SECONDARY EDUCATION

The world of secondary education was equally monochrome. Almost all institutions providing secondary education were church controlled and owned. It is true that many of these were excellent academies staffed by dedicated educators who received little reward beyond hoping to see their protégés penetrate to the upper echelons of society – a perfectly laudable ambition. In the words of one distinguished alumnus speaking of a Jesuit academy, 'we were expected to lead in society'.[123]

They were however, in 1950, unlikely to side with the Minister for Health and lead in a direction in which the Bishops did not want to go.

TERTIARY EDUCATION

With the exception of Trinity College the Catholic Church had, vicariously, almost complete control of the universities.

There was no better example of the manner in which Maynooth exercised such vicarious control than that of Alfred O'Rahilly, President of University College Cork. Around this time he wrote the following in a handwritten memorandum to the Archbishop of Dublin, John Charles McQuaid.[124] Clearly they were birds of a very conservative Catholic feather.

> I am convinced that in education and in health services, the Government's policy is by public funds to compete successfully with voluntary schools and hospitals, to cause slow financial strangulation of these latter in favour of State institutions (vocational schools and public hospitals). In ultimate this means usurpation of the Family by the State. There will be no open attacks, no immediately effective measures. There will be lip service to Catholic social principles, specious professions of goodwill, covering up and concealing the sinister financial pressure. In my opinion the establishment of Vocational Schools and the Health Act are the two

greatest blows which Catholic social principles have received in this country.

It would have been acceptable for O'Rahilly to hold such views as a private citizen. He was, however, articulating his essentially sectarian view as leader of a major publicly funded university. He was furthermore able to impose his Catholic mores on the campus of what purported to be a liberal educational institution. This effect endured some time after his departure as exemplified by the stultifying Medical Ethics course as previously discussed.

There is no mention in O'Rahilly's missive of the deplorable state of the nation's health nor of the parlous state of his own and other medical schools. He holds the strange view that the State should not act 'in favour of State institutions' – its own institutions. Then comes the extraordinary proposition that he himself might be appointed by the Hierarchy as what later came to be known as a 'spin doctor', for the views of the conservative right.

> May I respectfully and confidentially make a suggestion to his Grace? To counter the continuous Government propaganda and the confusion in the minds of our people, a very small and private advisory body would be very useful. A person like me could then be equipped and advised, or an anonymous encouragement could be given to weekly or daily papers. At the moment we need factually fortified statements about our secondary schools and our Catholic hospitals.

O'Rahilly is proposing a campaign of disinformation, a dirty tricks department. While by the time this was written Noël Browne had departed the scene (1954), it exemplifies well the monolithic Catholic establishment against which it had been futile for him to struggle.

Cavalry in a Bog

While the timing of Noël Browne's confrontation with the Bishops was inauspicious, the issue on which they clashed was for him catastrophic.

While the Catholic Church in many other countries was happy to articulate its quixotic approach to all matters sexual and procreative, it was beginning to lighten up somewhat and look with a little less censure on the transgressions of its followers in such matters.[125] Not so in Ireland. On all such matters in Ireland the Hierarchy were possessed by a paranoia of Kremlin proportions. With what would seem to be a very low opinion of the proclivities of their flock, they sought to throw a wet blanket over the national libido. For those who disagree with this analysis, or choose to disremember, that wet blanket extended to many other areas not least arts and literature. Writers of the greatest distinction who did not share Their Lordships asexual view of Ireland were censored, had their work placed on 'the Index',[126] and were driven out to places of toleration. Only eight years had passed since the book burning of Gougane Barra.[127]

In addition to the religious fervour militating against any possibility of resistance to the Bishops, there are reasons to wonder if in fact de Valera might have stood up to them with more backbone than the incoming Taoiseach on whose desk the problem now rested. It should be remembered that de Valera had sidestepped the issue when his Government introduced the 1947 Health Act to which the Bishops took exception.

Never has the long finger, applied to an identical issue, delivered such contrasting outcomes to Taoisigh in Irish politics: it saved de Valera from a conflict with the Bishops and landed Costello in one. De Valera procrastinated until overtaken by a general election which he lost. The incendiary issue was then dumped in the lap of the new Costello Government

The Archbishop was known to consider John A. Costello a much softer touch than de Valera and later, when the Mother and Child Scheme was done and dusted, he was known to give thanks that he had been dealing with the former and not the latter. The Archbishop's contrasting affections for the two leaders are exemplified by a vignette related to the rather prosaic matter of petrol supplies in times of scarcity. His favourite Taoiseach, Costello, back in Government, bent regulations during the subsequent Suez crisis (1956), when the citizen's tank was empty, to see to it that His Grace in Drumcondra could – 'unlike the rest of men' – continue motoring. This, His Grace observed with acidity, was 'a consideration which was not shown me during the war' – that is, World War II, when, of course, de Valera was manning the pumps.

While nobody doubts that de Valera was anything but a full blooded politician, Costello is considered by some to have been a reluctant one. In any case, while procrastination had extricated de Valera from the dangers of Episcopal confrontation in 1947, it had the opposite effect for Costello and pitched him into a full blown crisis with the Bishops and his Minister for Health.

On the face of it, an observer, even one of some paranoia, might expect to find little of taboo in a public health scheme to improve the appalling standards endured by the mothers and children of the nation. However, anything even vaguely related to 'sex relations, chastity and marriage', the triad set out in the 'Ferns' letter, should have been anticipated as an irresistible lure for the Hierarchy. And so it came to pass. The Archbishop rose to the lure as a trout in a western lake to the mayfly. The Minister had, like a poor general, blundered with his cavalry into a bog. The medical establishment, regarding him as one of their own gone bad, now knew that the quagmire would consume him. Furthermore, they must have rejoiced that the exemplary manner of his destruction would consolidate their position and serve as a salutary lesson in *realpolitik* for a generation of politicians to come.

The medical *agents provocateurs* could now relax in the knowledge that their campaign of obstruction would be pressed home by the Archbishop with much greater effect than they could bring to bear on their own.

13

BURNING BRIDGES

The Taoiseach's letter to Noël Browne, as discussed previously, when he finally woke up to the seriousness of his predicament, was dated 21 March 1951. Such was its content and import that a Minister of more political nous, on receipt of such a missive from his boss, would take pause and at the very least sleep on it before shooting off a vitriolic shaft in reply. Such, however, was not the way of this most impolitic of Ministers who, before the sun set, reached for his quill and shot off a most incendiary and bridge-burning riposte.

> I should have thought it unnecessary to point out that from the beginning it has been my concern to see that the Mother and Child Scheme contained nothing contrary to Catholic moral teaching.

This opening shot was bordering on the reckless. The tone suggests that he wonders if the Taoiseach, a man of intellectual accomplishment well used to thinking on his feet, was so dumb as to be unable to grasp his Minister's position. The Minister therefore must vouchsafe to 'point out' to him that which he should have been able to work out for himself.

Again, we have the matter of 'Catholic moral teaching' on which the Minister has educated himself and feels on solid ground. The Taoiseach harboured no theological pretensions and would pass it on to McQuaid. The Minister is baiting a trap in order to induce the Archbishop to come out on whether a fundamental moral issue was involved. If the Archbishop went for the bait the Minister would then, with reasoned argument, demolish him. Thus the Minister would hoist the Archbishop by his own theological petard.

The wily old fox in Drumcondra, however, trapped by his own hubris, knew there was no theological flaw in the scheme. Twice the Minister's age and ten times his match in native cunning and worldliness, and mindful that any theological gaffe would undermine his position, he was unlikely to fall for this ploy. The Archbishop after all existed on a higher, more celestial plane than the upstart Minister doctor dabbling in theology. He was God's Minister and in the Ireland of 1950, more than a match for anyone, Minister or otherwise, who merely derived his mandate from the people. He regarded politicians, heretofore compliant but now becoming irksome, as mere transients in his world of millennial permanence.

Noël Browne's next sentence should give pause to the many who extol him and would be his hagiographers.

> I hope I need not assure you that as a Catholic I will unhesitatingly and immediately accept any pronouncement from the Hierarchy as to what is Catholic moral teaching in this matter.

It has become fashionable with the passage of time, and the progressive atrophy of the Catholic Church in Ireland, to portray Noël Browne as one who ferociously stood out against it in its heyday. In this sentence, however, he is ardently professing his Catholicism and indeed appears somewhat affronted that his bona fides with regard to obedience to Bishops might be regarded as in any way suspect. He then lets the cat out of the bag completely. He points out to the Taoiseach that he will 'unhesitatingly and immediately', as the elected Minister for Health, sublimate the interests of the State to 'any pronouncement from the Hierarchy as to what is Catholic moral teaching'. In this pronouncement, alas, he reveals himself, at this time, to be little different to other elements of the Church–State complex in acknowledging the primacy of the former over the latter. The Minister was, in spite of everything, proving to be, as St Luke[128] might put it, 'as the rest of men'.

The obsequiousness of these remarks must have caused Noël Browne some discomfiture as the subsequent revisionism, which would portray him as a stout resistor of Bishops, took hold. He was still a convinced Catholic at this time. His mauling by the Bishops, however, would embitter the man and, in spite of the Jesuitical boasts, he would shake off his chains and, in the manner of all apostates, come to despise the organisation that had nurtured him.

And then yet again, through the Taoiseach, he taunts the Bishops:

> I am not satisfied that the Hierarchy are opposed to the scheme on grounds of faith and morals.

He is in effect saying to them, you are against the scheme for various worldly reasons but these have nothing to do with faith and morals. Shame on you.

THEIR LORDSHIPS ARE NOT SATISFIED

The complete breakdown of trust and working relationship between the Taoiseach and his Minister for Health is now apparent. Noël Browne continues to insist that the Taoiseach provide him with reasons why his Scheme is not being approved:

> I note that you have not addressed yourself to any of these reasons.

The reason, however, is singular, is known to all, and resides in Drumcondra.

The Minister then goes on to make clear his view that the Taoiseach is behaving duplicitously:

> ... following upon your interview with His Grace the
> Archbishop of Dublin on October 12th 1950 you assured
> me that His Grace and Their Lordships of Ferns and
> Galway were satisfied.

This is a most serious and damning allegation. The Taoiseach, John A. Costello, is generally represented by historians as having been an honourable man. If he had told his Minister, as stated above, that the triumvirate were 'satisfied' and then recanted without explanation, abandoning his Minister, the word honourable seems less appropriate. It boils down – as does much during this narrative – to a matter of whom one believes. The case, however, supporting the Minister's veracity, and indeed suggesting the Taoiseach's duplicity, is fortified by their respective actions. The Minister felt that he could make his case by immediately publishing the relevant correspondence. The Taoiseach had nothing so convincing to offer. Most of what passed on what he admitted to be the 'many occasions' on which he discussed the issue with the Archbishop, never saw the light of day.

As this letter progresses it becomes increasingly rancorous and meandering and abandons all pretence at the deference which might normally be expected, and would be no more than good manners, when a Minister addressed his Taoiseach. Noël Browne has lost his cool and is now in self-destruct mode.

Regarding the infamous letter from the Bishop of Ferns to the Taoiseach (10 October 1950) and the reply which Noël Browne had immediately crafted for forwarding by the Taoiseach but which lay neglected on the latter's desk for many months the Minister comments bitterly:

> I was under the impression that you had sent it as a reply
> to the letter of His Lordship the Bishop of Ferns and I
> was horrified to learn for the first time only a few days
> ago that you had never sent it.

The Minister for Health had indeed good reason to be 'horrified' to realise that, between 10 October 1950 and 21 March 1951, while he was ploughing ahead with his plans, the Taoiseach had in fact not received 'approval' from Drumcondra. Noël Browne would have us believe – and his letter in this regard is a matter of public record – that he was not aware of the continuing impasse. The Minister was a man of action and he was incredulous that the Head of Government could allow such drift.

While the Minister's training in medicine, augmented by his intense personality, had made him a man of action, his boss the Taoiseach had been trained as a barrister. The barrister's *métier* is to tease things out with words, and indeed with legal argument, in the hope that a satisfactory solution will emerge. It would, therefore, be in the very nature of such a man, and particularly as in this instance a procrastinating man, to 'let the hare sit'. It would be contrary to all his instincts to respond reflexly and petulantly as his Minister was increasingly doing. The hare was by now, however, sitting for many months and would not for much longer be restrained.

THE HOUNDS OF GOD

Those diminishing few who would admit to familiarity with such country pursuits will understand the metaphor of the hare. In his grassy forum, although discovered by the beater, he holds tough. The beater lets him sit until the hounds are optimally deployed for the chase. When, eventually, the long-legged athletic beast bolts, all hell breaks loose. With the hounds of man in pursuit of a country Sunday afternoon, happily the hare almost always escaped – blood sport without blood. When the hounds of God,[129] took pursuit of a politician in Ireland in 1950, however, it was a real blood sport, and blood they would have and the Taoiseach knew it.

The hounds of God were now on the Minister for Health, and they would hunt him to destruction.

The Minister continues to heap censure on the Taoiseach. Having previously said that the Bishops were 'satisfied' after the Minister met them, he is 'now' saying that they were not. He accuses the Taoiseach of being 'inconsistent'. To this Minister inconsistency was anathema. The Taoiseach, however, was of a different background and temperament. It was normal for him as a barrister to bend before the prevailing wind of fact and fiction which blew through his favourite stamping ground in the Four Courts, and to vary his position in the light of all that was coming at him. This flexibility was a positive attribute in Court or Parliament, and would have been regarded as normal, and indeed as honourable, by the Taoiseach. This was a Minister for Health, however, who would prefer to snap in the wind rather than bend with it and he was uncomprehending of the Taoiseach's pragmatism.

Then he makes an accusation:

> ... you allowed the scheme to develop without ever suggesting that the objection of His Grace the Archbishop of Dublin and their Lordships of Ferns and Galway were still unresolved

> ... you never discussed that aspect of the matter with me or questioned me about it until the 14th instant.

During all of this time while the Taoiseach had 'allowed the scheme to develop', he had, by his own admission, many informal meetings with the Archbishop while ignoring his Minister. While it is clear that the Taoiseach was at this time under great pressure, this was no way to conduct government business.

It is striking, particularly from the perspective of the twenty-first century, that all parties to the correspondence, including Noël Browne, tacitly accepted one verity – Their Lordships must be 'satisfied'.

THE MEANS TEST

While the Taoiseach was bypassing the Minister for Health in his discussions with the Archbishop, he was likewise bypassing and ignoring him by having discussions with the Irish Medical Association. Predictably, these latter discussions revolved not around any spurious matter of faith and morals as with the Bishops. The IMA, although they would protest otherwise, were concerned about money. The IMA wanted the application of a means test to the new scheme. Dáil Éireann had, however, passed the new scheme without a means test. There was general agreement, with the exception of the Bishops and doctors, that the scheme, if means tested, would not achieve its potential. In this regard the IMA, in material circulated to members, quoted the Taoiseach as telling them:

> ... neither the Dail nor Senate would approve any amendment of the Act or Regulations which would envisage the omission of a free service for all.

Now the means test becomes fundamental to the entire enterprise. The Minister had stated himself prepared to 'satisfy' the Bishops on all the other issues they had raised. He had 'compromised on the offending clauses' with regard to the education of women. He would 'reconsider these clauses'. He was prepared even to accept that the Hierarchy could 'submit their own' clauses covering areas about which they had anxiety. With these concessions any legitimate moral objection, as distinct from a spurious one, was removed. Another blocking issue must be found: one on which the Minister would not yield.

The only sticking point now for the Minister was that the scheme must be completely free-for-all. He would give the Bishops anything they wanted but he would make his stand on the no means test principle – the principle of universality. A means test would undermine the potential and *raison d'être* of the scheme. It would retain the 'mark of the Poor Law'.

The Minister is in effect saying that The Taoiseach previously had no issue with the absence of a means test but now, having been got at, was abandoning that position and abandoning his Minister to boot. The situation was now running out of control. One wonders if the Hierarchy by this time might have begun to feel like the wife manipulated Macbeth. They were however in absurdity 'stepped in so far ... returning were as tedious as go o'er'.[130] And all the while, in the 'Squares and the Crescents',[131] with God's main man in Ireland homing in on their target like military drone remotely controlled, there was much rejoicing.

THE HOUR IS LATE

The hour was indeed late for the Minister for Health. He is, in addition, to a considerable extent in denial and is deluding himself on two counts.

> It seems strange that at this late hour when the discussions with the Irish Medical Association have reached a crucial point that you advance as the only objection to the Scheme the one which of all possible objections – namely the supposed opposition of the Hierarchy, should have first been satisfactorily disposed of.

Firstly, The Minister was deluding himself that he had 'satisfactorily disposed of' Their Lordships objections at the infamous meeting with the three Bishops many months before. Whether or not the Episcopal triumvirate were 'satisfied' at that meeting is moot and has been much discussed earlier. What is clear is that they certainly are not 'satisfied' now, months later, and while the dogs in the street knew this, the Minister affects a less than credible surprise.

Secondly, while he must surely know now that his scheme is doomed, he deludes himself that he almost had it in the bag with the Irish Medical Association, but for the meddling of the Catholic Hierarchy. Nothing could be further from the truth.

The doyens of medicine, who controlled opinion in the doctor's union, were as implacable as ever and were, in addition, now cocksure having recruited the unstoppable Archbishop of Dublin as their patsy: as Noël Browne put it in his memoir, they had become 'intransigent'. For the Minister to suggest that his discussions with the IMA had reached 'a crucial point' rings hollow. The talks had reached an impasse and, while the Archbishop continued to play at full back on the doctor's team, their goal was well guarded and they had no reason to give ground.

The Minister states and readily concedes that the Bishops' objections:

> Should first have been satisfactorily disposed of before any steps were taken in furtherance of the Mother and Child Scheme.

Of 'all possible objections' to anything new, which might have confronted politicians of the day that which most terrified them was any hint of 'opposition of the Hierarchy'. In fact the Minister for Health is suggesting that, of all the potential impediments to new and progressive legislation, none mattered as much as getting the nod from Their Lordships. An unstable cabinet kaleidoscopic in spectrum, unreliable deputies of unpredictable voting, perpetual budget challenges, the economy in the doldrums, the IRA still smouldering – all of these and many other political banana skins were as nothing compared to the potential catastrophe of a raised eyebrow in Drumcondra.

This conceded to the Hierarchy the *de facto* status of lawmakers.

14

Taoiseach Washes His Hands

Events, with their capacity, famously, to disrupt the orderly affairs of government,[132] were now gathering pace and the whole descent into disaster had taken on an unstoppable momentum. The Taoiseach, having sat on the fence for many months – a posture which historically had served him well – is now replying to his increasingly truculent Minister by return. John Costello had perhaps realised that the tectonic speed of the Irish legal process, to which he was accustomed and of which he was an arch exponent, does not work so well when Government is smitten by 'events', and that all the while during which he has been dithering, tension has been gathering towards an inevitable seismic upheaval which will now pull the house down upon him.

Earthquakes of the seismic variety are of course unknown in Ireland. Indeed, by the middle of the twentieth century Episcopal eruptions – notwithstanding the quixotic follies of the Bishop of Galway – had also become rare and almost redundant. Their Lordships bestrode the land like ayatollahs, and so compliant was the population and the body politic that the mere threat of eruption was sufficient to keep order and the crozier could remain in its holster.

The new and youthful Minister for Health, however, now seemed to be having some difficulty understanding Their Catholic Lordships' standing orders to Government. To reassert their authority Their Lordships needed to administer to the Minister a booster dose of Episcopal chastisement in order to awaken the sleeping phagocytes[133] to the danger of invasion by what the IMA called 'the cancer of socialised medicine'. It was regarded as normal, in a strange inversion of roles, that the elected Government should cede to the unelected its prerogatives in any area of the Hierarchy's choosing.

The head of Government in a Republic must separate his private beliefs from his public duties and can do so without detriment to the former. If unable or unprepared to do this he should not accept the office. This principle was exemplified *par excellence* by the thirty-ninth President of the United States, Jimmy Carter, who, although privately a devout Christian and opposed to abortion, publicly gave assent to the Roe versus Wade Bill legalising that procedure. Indeed, he did so in the face of virulent, and on occasions violent, opposition from the religious right.

The Taoiseach of 1950, John A. Costello, and his cabinet were incapable of such intellectual agility. The consequences for development of the Health Services were catastrophic and enduring: elite vested interests in medicine and Church continued to rule while the public interest played second fiddle. Indeed, almost a quarter of a century later not a lot had changed when a later Taoiseach[134] voted against his own Government on a contraception bill. At that time, when the very existence of the State was threatened by violent subversives, its politicians still considered the Bishops a greater danger. The accoutrements of contraception were a bigger threat to the nation than the paraphernalia of bomb making.

The booster dose of 1951 had worked well.

And now Noël Browne, whose legitimate powers had been usurped by Bishops and senior doctors, was, when he attempted to recoup those powers, himself branded as the usurper.

The Taoiseach, at last energised, is now replying to his Minister by return. He does not, however, provide any of the reasons and explanations which the Minister has been demanding. He washes his hands with the capitulation, 'it is for the Hierarchy alone to say whether or no the scheme contained anything contrary to Catholic moral teaching'.

The correspondence between the Taoiseach and his Minister has now degenerated into a squabble and during squabbles excuses abound. John A. Costello, accustomed as a barrister to dealing with the excuses and explanations of others, is now obliged to offer some on his own behalf.

The Taoiseach explains his delay in dealing with the correspondence from the Bishop of Ferns:

> ... my actions in this matter have been ... entirely actuated by what I conceived to be a friendly desire to help a colleague.

The best way to have helped his Minister however would have been to support him in his resistance to the Bishops. This, however, was not what he meant by 'help'. It was rather that he wished to enlighten the Minister as to the folly of continuing his attempt to introduce measures to improve the health service in the face of resistance from the Bishops. What he wished to do was not so much to help his Minister but rather to rehabilitate him. Rehabilitation – a word much loved by totalitarian regimes of the time – implied some malady of mind or body. The Minister was suffering from a bad case of Bishop Resistance Syndrome – usually a fatal affliction for an Irish politician – and, failing urgent rehabilitation, would succumb.

During this rehabilitative process the Minister must – and Noël Browne was singularly unpromising material for such a *volte face* – completely purge himself of the deviant notion that Bishops should not have the final say in the healthcare policy of the nation.

Only a man accustomed to turning meaning on its head in the courts could have the gall to speak of 'my actions' when, for close on six months, he had been paralysed in the face of the gathering storm and had done exactly nothing. Perhaps he hoped that a cooling off period would cause either the Archbishop or the Minister for Health to relent. This, however, is never a likely outcome 'when two strong men stand face to face'.[135]

Having failed to join his contemporaries in their battle to wrest Ireland from the British Empire, the Taoiseach was even less likely to attempt to prise it away from an altogether more formidable force – the Irish Catholic Bishops. In the face of contrary argument from his Minister a lawyer like the Taoiseach might be expected to fall back upon his stock and trade of reasoned argument. Hobbled by the Bishops, however, and bereft of material for such argument, he resorts to the less credible device of indignation.

> I take it somewhat amiss to find misconstrued my endeavours to have the objection to the Scheme, which had been advanced on behalf of the Hierarchy, satisfactorily resolved.

An argument supported only by indignation is already lost.

The Taoiseach then proceeds further to erode his credibility by offering more excuses:

> In the hope that these objections could be satisfactorily disposed of I refrained from replying to the letter from His Lordship the Bishop of Ferns.

Taoiseach John A. Costello wanted the Hierarchical objections satisfactorily resolved. But resolution of such disputes requires bilateral discussion. The Archbishop of Dublin, John Charles McQuaid, however, was not a bilateral man. His idea of bilateral discussion was to summon the Minister to his presence, outline his position, dismiss the Minister, and then undermine him by going behind his back to the Taoiseach. This behind the back discussion is amply confirmed by the following statement from the Taoiseach:

> I explained to His Grace the Archbishop of Dublin my reasons for so refraining and he communicated these to the Hierarchy

The Taoiseach concludes his letter in the tone of father confessor:

> I need hardly say that I accept unreservedly your statement that you would abide by any pronouncement from the Hierarchy as to what is Catholic moral teaching in reference to this matter.

Here we have the Prime Minister of a Republic who is prepared to act as a vigilante for the Catholic Church. He will see to it that his Ministers, and particularly the incumbent of the Department of Health, do not upset the comfortable apple cart of the *Pax Romana*.[136] The vigilante is much reassured that his difficult Minister for Health, although politically errant, is religiously sound. On foot of this reassurance therefore he is prepared to mollify his tone and act as father confessor.

The Minister for Health, however, was an unpromising penitent. Absolution for a sin that he did not commit – for he knew that the 'moral' argument was bogus – was never going to turn him. The Taoiseach is at pains to reassure his Minister that, whatever their disagreements, whatever damage the Minister's schemes might inflict on the affairs of State and Government, whatever he might think of the man and his character, he did not accuse him of that most heinous of all crimes in the Ireland of 1950 – disobedience to Bishops.

One is tempted to ponder to what extent, if at all, these two men – the Taoiseach and the Minister for Health – were now prepared to sit down together and discuss their mutual problem which was about to consume them both.

Certainly the Taoiseach was, by all accounts, an affable and genial man and, as mentioned earlier, an avoider of confrontation – this latter tendency perhaps the cause of his undoing in the present *imbroglio*. He was also well accustomed, on the steps of the Four Courts or inside, to last minute conflict resolution by discussion and compromise. When it came to the diktats of authoritarian Catholicism, however, there was to be no compromise: he was subservient in all things to the Episcopal dictation. Indeed, on taking office he was at pains to reassure the Pope that in governing the Irish Republic he was prepared to 'repose at the feet of Your Holiness the assurance of our filial loyalty and devotion.'

Noël Browne was, by contrast, with regard to personality, attitude and political creed, everything that his Taoiseach was not. That which the Taoiseach considered virtuous – political subservience to the Church – the Minister for Health came to despise. That upon which the Minister was insisting – that the Archbishop of Dublin was out of order in his meddling – was profane to the Taoiseach. East was east and west was west, or perhaps more appropriately, left was left and right was right, and never the twain would meet – a self-destruct mechanism inherent in all coalition Governments in Ireland.

The now daily exchange of correspondence between Taoiseach and Minister suggests that whatever verbal dialogue the twain had before had now ceased. In schoolyard parlance – and their behaviour was now indeed infantile – they were just not talking. For separated lovers daily correspondence replete with sweet nothings has long been known to fan the flames of desire resulting in eventual successful cohabitation. In pursuit of political cohabitation, however, the formula is less proven. Furthermore, while the correspondence between the two is now punctuated by a great many nothings, these alas are predominantly of the bitter kind. Bitter nothings are much less conducive to cohabitation than sweet nothings.

It is also apparent from the letter that the scheme, approved by cabinet, and advanced as Government policy, is now, with some measure of dishonour, being disowned by the Taoiseach. He does not speak of the scheme as Government policy but rather, with pejorative undertones, as 'the Mother and Child Scheme as outlined by you'. He is in effect saying your scheme is an unwanted baby and we are leaving you holding it. The Taoiseach, having sat on his hands for months, is now in biblical fashion, washing them of this tainted scheme and of his troublesome Minister. He must trim his sails to the new wind.

The wind to which the Taoiseach was now busily adjusting his sails was a chill northerly one blowing down from Drumcondra. This wind was not at all new and had been safely navigated for more than a century, first by the British administration which had found the Church a useful proxy for controlling seditious elements, and following their departure, by the new State. True, there had been occasional inconvenient gusts but nothing as tempestuous as the squall which the Archbishop now threatened to unleash on the ever increasingly absurd non-issue of the means test, the absence of which he was now representing as a threat to faith and morals. The northerly wind, previously steady, was becoming unpredictable and the Taoiseach knew that, unless he reefed in some sail, a gust would come out of Drumcondra to capsize him. He must therefore now move on his Minister. Noël Browne was indeed, in real life, an accomplished sailor. He was however alas less competent at managing the metaphoric Episcopal wind than the real meteorological one – the former altogether more dangerous.

Also, the Taoiseach at this time is again showing himself to be maladroit at the political art. He has allowed himself to be manoeuvred into a position whereby he will be damned if he does and damned if he does not. He can now give in to the Bishops or give in to his Minister. If he gives in to the Bishops the Minister will go, and not quietly. It should be remembered that the Minister was a master of publicity and a classical practitioner of 'pork barrel' politics, and his populist ideas chimed with the public (or at least with the less well off majority). After his ouster the Minister, difficult though he might have been in cabinet, would be altogether more so outside of it. He would now be outside the tent creating much nuisance. In this event the Government was unlikely to survive.

The alternative scenario was that the Taoiseach – and this would run counter to all that we have observed about him – would stand his ground and face down the Bishops. Facing down Bishops in the Ireland of 1950 was a singularly unappetising prospect which few who did not live through those times would understand today. For a Taoiseach in particular to engage in such an adventure, especially when there was a whiff of 'faith and morals' in the air, would be rash indeed and might amount to the first of the then much touted 'seven deadly sins' – pride. The fate of the arch offender in this area, Lucifer, was much preached in Ireland. The Taoiseach knew that if he did not buckle, the Bishops would rouse the country against him and he would be likewise cast down. Lucifer indeed, although rarely given credit for it, was a rather principled fellow – 'better to reign in hell than serve in heaven'.[137] The Taoiseach, however, not like Lucifer afflicted by pride, would as a result of his subservience to the Bishops end up with the worst of both worlds – he would serve in hell.

And yet these two options – to reign or to serve – were not mutually exclusive. The Taoiseach was a daily Mass-goer where he doubtless listened to the Gospels. It is surprising that he did not use his acknowledged advocacy skills to press this scriptural wisdom into greater service in his dealing with the Archbishop. The Gospels were after all the stock in trade of the latter. What better man to quote on the contentious issue of the relations between Church and State than Jesus Christ himself. What better way to floor a Bishop, or indeed and

Archbishop, than to counter his spoof with the very words of the founder of Christianity. If St Matthew is to be believed, and it would be odd for an Archbishop to reject him, Jesus offered a way out of the impasse: 'Render unto Caesar the things that are Caesar's and to God the things that are God's'. Certainly Jesus, who did not have a public relations entourage to tell him what to say, spontaneously delivered himself of a fine piece of equivocation to confound his detractors. The devout Taoiseach would without doubt have been familiar with this neat piece of scriptural obfuscation. Furthermore, politicians are by definition obfuscators, and certainly nobody reaches the Taoiseach's office without having mastered that art. In addition to his ability to obfuscate in Parliament, which is of course *de rigueur* for a head of Government, he was a legendary exponent of that faculty at the Bar. Yet he missed this great opportunity to hoist the Archbishop by his own petard.

Sadly, the Taoiseach's intellectual machinery, normally well lubricated, seized up entirely when confronted by Episcopal authority and, abandoning his Republic, he was reduced to a supine state of obeisance.

Noël Browne replied to the Taoiseach promptly on 24 March 1951 enclosing his final explanatory memorandum:

> I am acting in accordance with the suggestion of His Grace the Archbishop of Dublin with whom I discussed the matter on 22nd March 1951. He appears to fully appreciate the extreme urgency of the serious situation which has developed within the cabinet and of its likely implications to its future. I would ask you to be good enough to forward without delay this memorandum for the early consideration and decision of the question contained therein.

The Taoiseach is reduced to a mere transmitter of documents.

There is menace in the Minister's letter. He speaks of 'implications' for the future of the cabinet and has seen to it that the Archbishop, and now the Taoiseach, understand these implications. He will have his way or bring a plague on both their houses.

The Minister, mindful of the Taoiseach's earlier procrastination, requests pointedly that his memorandum should be forwarded to the Hierarchy 'without delay'. There is little in his references to Bishops at this time of the heroic persona which would later become his motif. Right now he meekly awaits 'the decision' of Their Lordships on this matter.

The Taoiseach promptly received the Minister's memorandum and sent it with a covering letter to the Hierarchy. As requested, he sent a copy of this covering letter to the Minister. This letter to the Bishop of Ferns, as secretary to the Hierarchy, is replete with the feudal subservience which characterised all Costello's communications with senior churchmen.

For those who would defend the intimacy of Church and State in post-independence Ireland, this letter (Appendix 2) should be required reading. It portrays a total, abject and unconditional surrender of the *Res Publica* to the unelected Princes of the Church. Rome rule it was indeed. Ulster Unionists, long trumpeting this canard, were again certain that they were 'right'. They had faithfully served an empire which was now, to their alarm, exhausted and preparing to fold its imperial tent right across the globe. The mother country could surely not now abandon them also to the tender mercies of the priest ridden south. The Taoiseach, by his subservience to the Bishops and to Rome, was following a course odious to Northern Unionists and thus serving to cement partition. Although avowedly anti-partitionist, he was doing more than most to perpetuate the division of Ireland.

It is confirmed here also that the infamous letter from the Secretary to the Hierarchy, the Bishop of Ferns, objecting to the Mother and Child Scheme, did not arrive with a tuppeny stamp in the regular post. The Taoiseach got the letter directly from 'His Grace of Dublin'. God's main man in Ireland delivered it himself – by hand. This demonstrative act, making it plain that Their Lordships meant business, would have had a salutary effect on the genuinely devout Taoiseach, and this is reflected in his letter.

There can be little doubt that the Taoiseach and his cabinet were giving 'anxious consideration' to the objections of the Hierarchy. Merely giving careful consideration, it would seem, might have been insufficient to convince Their Lordships that their message had got through. While the Taoiseach himself may have had some genuine fear of hellfire and damnation, there is little doubt that his colleagues in government were exercised by the less nebulous prospect of being kicked out of office.

Not for the first time the Taoiseach is putting distance between himself and his Minister for Health. Increasingly, the problem Mother and Child Scheme is portrayed as being 'advocated by the Minister for Health' rather than by the Government, and emphatically not by the head of Government. What now of collective cabinet responsibility? The question of over-ruling 'the objections of the Hierarchy' was, clearly, never considered. Ireland, North and South, would have been better served if the Taoiseach had stood by his Minister and by the collective decision already taken, and forced the scheme through.

It is symptomatic of the conspiratorial shenanigans that we know little, from the official record, of the 'many occasions' on which these matters were discussed between the Taoiseach and Archbishop. Clearly it was the view of both that what the public did not know would not bother them. The letter was, of course, written in the expectation that it would not see the light of day for a generation. The Taoiseach, even if he did not respect the electorate, had plenty reason to fear them. The Archbishop neither respected nor feared. While clearly not affecting the infallibility of his boss in Rome he did feel omniscient – a good second. But the Minister for Health had asked for, and got from the Taoiseach, a copy of the incendiary letter and it was smouldering in his files and would burst forth in a great conflagration long before its time.

PUGIN'S ARCH

In mid-twentieth century Ireland the 'standing committee' of the Catholic Hierarchy, to which Noël Browne's memorandum, explaining his scheme, was now making its circuitous way 'for an early decision', was indeed a formidable beast.

When, particularly after one of their plenary sessions, their assembled Lordships sallied forth through Pugin's[138] arch at Maynooth in full regalia the reportage of a compliant, indeed censored, press became a set-piece. They appeared very much of the world. Doubtless there were some good and saintly men amongst them but under the autocratic Archbishop McQuaid their genius was 'rebuked as it is said Mark Anthony's was by Caesar's'.[139] To this observer, although then just a boy, they did not seem like the kind of fellows who would wash the feet of their inferiors as Jesus had done.

From Their Lordship's Rampant, the Minister's memorandum would receive a frosty reception.

The Government was awaiting not the opinion, not the view, not even the advice – 'the decision'. The future structure of the Irish health service awaited a 'decision' from Maynooth. Even at the remove of six decades this is extraordinarily supine: grist to the mill of certain northern demagogue preachers them emerging.

There is a comic element to the northern enigma germane to the said Bishops.

The island of Ireland is over endowed with no less than twenty-six dioceses including four archdioceses. Three of these dioceses, along with the Archdioceses of Armagh, straddle the border. A bishop of such a straddling dioceses was expected to accept a total National Health Service in the northern part (British jurisdiction) of his fief, while at the same time resisting to the death the merest increment of such a service in the southern part (Irish jurisdiction). And to compound this unfortunate man's discomfiture, he was supposed to accept this Catch-22 absurdity[140] on the grounds of faith and morals.

Then from the Taoiseach comes an apologia for his failure to face up to the issue earlier. This, he explains, was perfectly acceptable behaviour because 'both His Grace of Dublin and I' agreed on that course.

In passing, it is interesting to observe the frequency with which the Taoiseach uses honorific titles in this letter (Appendix 2): the words Grace and Lordship appear (in aggregate) no less than twelve times – heady language indeed for the Prime Minister of a Republic which affected disdain for such titles, and which has always shied away from any honours system for worthy lay contributors to society.

Unashamedly, the Taoiseach writes that the Minister for Health had been 'warned' by the Archbishop. He is resorting now, not to the circumlocutions of the courtroom, but to the vulgarity of the football field. The Minister had been guilty of a reckless tackle upon the Hierarchy and the referee above in Drumcondra had waved the yellow card. He had let it be known that the crozier was already out and swinging. One more foul tackle on Team Hierarchy and the red card, itching in the soutane pocket, would be out and flashing.

The passivity of the Taoiseach is striking. He has sent the matter for 'decision', if we may continue the sporting metaphor albeit in a different code, 'upstairs'. 'His Grace of Dublin' was, like the television match referee at Lansdowne Road or Thomond Park, all powerful. Everybody waited with trepidation, as at a major rugby match, or indeed in the Roman Coliseum, for the thumbs up or down.

The irony of the Archbishop of Dublin being good enough to keep the Taoiseach 'accurately informed' on what was primarily a political matter is apparently lost on the Taoiseach. There is also the implication that – communication having broken down between them – the Minister is not keeping his Taoiseach 'adequately informed'.

And now for the final debasement of the institutions of the State. The proposed healthcare measure is to be placed, for the thumbs up or down, not before the elected House of Parliament, but rather 'on the agenda of the forthcoming meeting of the Hierarchy'. To compound the absurdity, and indeed the impropriety, the request to place the item on the agenda is coming not from the Archbishop but from the Taoiseach, who is doing his bidding: the Archbishop has 'kindly agreed' that the Taoiseach should 'request Your Lordship the Most reverend Secretary' to put the Minister's memorandum on the agenda.

15

THE LETTER NOT WRITTEN

W e might here indulge in the composition of an imaginary letter which a more vertebrate Taoiseach might have sent to the Archbishop during the Mother and Child *imbroglio*. Such a letter was never sent. The thoughts contained therein were never articulated. The Church–medical conspiracy ensured that the Health Service would remain ideologically hobbled.

Dear Archbishop,

Let us consider our respective positions in the present difficulty. I think it is fair to say that we are both followers of Jesus Christ. You however being full time at it have a position of advantage in interpreting the Scriptures. My own position on such matters, since I am fully exercised in running a small but truculent country and in holding together a most combustible cabinet, is not to engage my mind on such profound questions but rather, in a general way, to be guided by the wisdom of Your Grace and Their Lordships, the professionals.

Your Grace will be aware that my background is in the law where we set great store on precedent and where accumulated wisdom is handed down for the betterment of others who come after. Indeed we have great tomes of law by which we live legally. I hope Your Grace will not take it amiss when I say that we regard these tomes as our 'Bible'. In their judgements Their Lordships – and I refer here to their secular Lordships of the bench – are most scrupulous in their researching of, familiarity with, and application of the contents of our 'Bible.' A judge who fails to apply precedent correctly may fall prey to clever barristers who will unmask his delinquency and have his judgement overturned in a higher court. As you can imagine our Lordships do not enjoy this kind of comeuppance and leave no tome unturned to avoid it. Again I beg your forbearance for my use of the word, but you might say that they adhere rigorously to our 'scriptures.'

This adherence to our 'scriptures' has enabled us to bring some credibility to the dispensing of legal judgements, and the sanction of appeal to a higher court enables us to restrain the solo run of the occasional maverick who finds his way onto the bench. The solo runner, I am sure you will agree, while cutting a great dash on the sports field, and frequently acclaimed by the populous, is the scourge of all disciplined organisations.

I would respectfully like to make it clear that the Minister for Health is not, as has been suggested, on a solo run with the Mother and Child Scheme. In his promotion of the scheme, to which you have taken some exception, he is merely the instrument of Government policy. The measures which he proposes were largely conceived by the previous Government (now in opposition), refined by us and approved by me and my cabinet colleagues as agreed Government policy. There is thus an overwhelming democratic mandate for the measure. But more of that later.

I come now to a matter of some delicacy, religious observance. My own belief is that this should be a private matter and that public displays are unbecoming. It is with some reluctance therefore, and only for the purpose of advancing my argument, that I offer that I am in frequent attendance and an avid listener to the Gospels. Mostly I agree with their gist and I often find their wisdom useful in dealing with a coalition cabinet which spans the political spectrum. For example to counter the demands of the left, with whom against all my instincts I am obliged to cohabit, I frequently deploy one of my favourites, 'The labourer in the vineyard.' It is a feature of my cabinet that although extremely heterogeneous in political orientation they are almost homogeneously of your

Grace's and my own religious persuasion and extremely receptive to biblical wisdom. Thus in matters of wage restraint, what constitutes a fair day's work and a fair day's pay, adherence to bargains and suchlike, I have found this tract extremely useful particularly with those members of my cabinet who made their way to greatness by way of trade unions.

Remarkably there is something for everybody in the Gospels and for my colleagues on the right, equally insatiable as those on the left, I sometimes resort to the parable of the Prodigal Son. Frankly my own inclination would be to abandon to his fate this feckless fellow who dissipated his inheritance in debauchery: Jesus however felt that he should be indulged and rehabilitated. This biblical advice of course, while it runs entirely counter to the instincts of my right wingers, is a great help to me in restraining them since they are, for the most part, in thrall to Catholic orthodoxy. Your Grace will see therefore that judicious application of this biblical cement has enabled me to hold together a very fractious Government – until now.

While it ill behoves a politician to cite scripture to an Archbishop I nevertheless take the liberty of raising the question of what is the correct relationship between Church and State or as St Matthew puts it, between God and Caesar. I am sure that Your Grace is familiar with the tract although your perspective on it, representing God so to speak as you do, will be quite different from my own since, for the purpose of the discussion I, as Taoiseach, might be considered to represent Caesar. Do you not think that this fine piece of equivocation, and by no less a figure than Jesus Christ, might offer us a way out of our difficulty?

Clearly Jesus was prepared to 'render unto Caesar the things that are Caesar's.' If Your Grace could just see your way to follow this ample precedent, and yield to me the prerogatives of State, we may yet extricate ourselves from this debacle which threatens to consume us both. For my own part I am happy, on behalf of the State, to 'render unto God the things that are God's,' but does the

Mother and Child Scheme belong to God or Caesar – there's the rub.

I myself, with my theologically untutored mind, have the greatest difficulty in understanding how a measure to improve the public health could be an affront to God. I am further confused as to how such a scheme might imperil the faith and morals of the nation. Is it possible that God approves of my Minister for Health and his Mother and Child Scheme? Could it be that God is not as preoccupied as the Hierarchy are by the Mother and Child affair and might be happy to 'render' it to the elected representatives of the people?

These of course are awkward thoughts for me, a devout Catholic, to express to you and I do so with reluctance and respect. Nevertheless might I venture to suggest that the increasing fusion of Church and State makes it impossible to run either efficiently? It is true that up to now we have muddled through but I hope you will not take it amiss if I suggest that the Church has had the better end of the bargain. Who could deny that on almost all occasions when the Bishops have dug their heels in, elected politicians have yielded?

There is another awkward thought that is troubling me and it relates to what some call 'the national question.' While I myself was not 'out' in 1916 or against the Black and Tans, nor did I participate in the odious civil war, I am dismayed by the continuing partition of Ireland and seek at all times to work peacefully towards its elimination. Towards this end therefore we should seek to bring about convergence of administrative structures in the two parts of Ireland. I have to state that Your Grace's posture towards the Mother and Child Scheme works towards divergence rather than convergence in the provision of medical services for the people. While I do not make so bold as to suggest that you are of partitionist mentality, I fear the position you have adopted will give succour to those who are.

Your Grace must be aware that, as in the rest of the United Kingdom, a full and comprehensive National Health Service regime now operates in Northern Ireland. By all accounts the citizens, Catholics and Protestants alike, are much enamoured of the service. Indeed that service is altogether more comprehensive than our proposed rather modest departure of the Mother and Child Scheme. Is it not surprising to you that the Catholic authorities in the North, where I am bound to observe that you are outranked by the Primate of all Ireland the Archbishop of Armagh, found this advance of the State into Medicine in no way repugnant. Not to put too fine a point on it, why is it that a big dose of 'socialised medicine' is easily digested by the Archbishop of Armagh while a much lesser dose, indeed one of homeopathic proportions, causes the Archbishop of Dublin to erupt? Surely that which threatens 'faith and morals' south of the border should be equally menacing north of it. Yet your ranking Archbishop colleague raised no objection while you threaten to bring down my Minister for Health and my Government.

Why is the introduction of a State medical service a matter for Caesar north of the border and for God south of it?

And here is another point. While not wishing to go behind your back, so to speak, I felt it incumbent on me to canvass the opinion of a number of your episcopal colleagues on this matter. It came as something of a surprise to me that not all agree with your position and some told me, might I say circumspectly and in the strictest confidence, that they see no connection between 'faith and morals' and the proposed Mother and Child Scheme.

I understand furthermore that among the foot soldiers of the Catholic clergy around the country, who interact with the public daily, there is considerable confusion regarding the rumoured position of the senior Hierarchy. I say 'rumoured' because of course we have, as much as possible, kept the public in the dark but this containment cannot be expected to last. Certainly my Minister for Health, if he is bested, will blow the gaffe immediately and completely. Those country clergymen, the backbone of the Church and indeed often of the communities in which they live, will be faced with the daunting task of explaining to believers why it is that a scheme to prevent maternal and infant mortality is against the will of a benign God.

When details of this whole unhappy business become public, as my Minister for Health will inevitably see to it that they do, Your Grace will have egg on his face. Church discipline will of course hold – una voce and all that. You will however, after some time, be the first of a new species in Ireland, a lame duck Bishop and with an increasingly sceptical public the species will proliferate. Worse awaits me however: I will be a dead duck Taoiseach.

I realise that Your Grace's father was a medical doctor and that consequently you may have an understandable empathy with the medical profession. I am likewise connected and indeed close to some of the most important doctors and professors in those important hospitals owned by the Church and governed by yourself. There is of course nothing wrong with any of this but I would ask you to consider that influential elements of the medical profession, with ready access to us both, are manipulating us for their own reasons. Put plainly they fear, in my opinion without justification, that the provision by the State gratis, of high quality medical services will eliminate their private practices and curtail their professional freedoms. The doctors have, with devilish cunning, recruited both of us, but you in particular, to their ignoble campaign.

When these facts become known the means test will be seen as the red herring of the century and Your Grace's reputation will forever carry a fishy taint. While our respective institutions of Church and politics will incur opprobrium, politicians are used to such censure, Bishops are not.

Time, Your Grace, is running out. My incendiary Minister's fuse is burning short and will soon cause him to explode: we will both suffer collateral damage. We must take immediate and decisive action to preserve the institutions of Church and politics, both of immense value to the people. Otherwise the effect for me will be the ousting of my Government. For your Church the effect will be more subtle and insidious, but ultimately more destructive. The people will no longer trust the Bishops and your authority will atrophy.

Might I return briefly to the awkward matter of consistency and the previously mentioned matter of the maverick judge? This awkward fellow, this solo runner of the bench, while an embarrassment to his colleagues, and erosive of confidence in the legal system, is subject to higher legal authority and this serves to control his eccentricity. Furthermore there is the added advantage that all his follies and foibles are acted out in full view of the public – justice seen to be done and all of that. The public might be amused or irate but at least they know what is happening. This, might I venture to offer, is in marked contrast to the secret deliberations of the Bishops who do not feel obliged to explain themselves publicly but rather seek to influence the functions of the State by secret diktats. Would Your Grace's laity not be better served, and your Church fortified, by a full and open explanation of why the Mother and Child Scheme is morally flawed? Or is it the case that Your Grace has no such explanation to offer? Certainly no such explanation appears in your correspondence with me or my Minister. Since the elected Government is in favour of the scheme, and the public will certainly welcome it, and certain Bishops see nothing wrong with it, and the Archbishop of Armagh has acquiesced in much more intrusive State health provision, I am bound to ask who is the maverick?

I propose therefore, in the event of Your Grace's continuing resistance, and in the absence of bilateral public debate, to authorise my Minister for Health to proceed immediately with the scheme and 'let slip the dogs of war'. The ensuing havoc will be no worse for me, and indeed will be more honourable than being seen to sacrifice a popular and hardworking Minister to the unexplained wishes of Bishops.

Dr Noël Browne, you will doubtless have noticed, is a formidable communicator. His humble background enables him to connect with the common people, as exemplified by his success at the polls. He is not likely to abide by Queensbury, or indeed Bishops' rules.

Once unleashed by me he will immediately go public and may, in order to pre-empt the Hierarchy, rehearse in the full light of day all that I have said in this letter and much more.

He will wax theological. He will ask why sauce for the goose in Newry is not sauce for the gander in Dundalk. He will talk of alienating Unionists and cementing partition. He will mix a heady cocktail of reason and rationale. Will Your Grace have the stomach for this? The credulity even of the Irish Catholic public has limits. Will Your Grace step out himself or will the Bishop of Ferns be deployed? Be assured that responding to the well thought out arguments of my Minister for Health is not something that his adversaries have found easy. The Bishop of Ferns is good enough on paper, especially with you at his elbow, but picking up the gauntlet which Noël Browne will throw down, is an unaccustomed challenge for Bishops.

Might I make so bold as to suggest a course of action by your good self which may yet deliver us both? I hope that you will see, when you reflect upon my proposal, that the prestige of the Church will be bolstered rather than battered by your decisive intervention as follows.

You must immediately make it known that the Catholic Hierarchy has no moral objection to the Mother and Child Scheme. This should be possible for you since the reservations which you have expressed to me and my Minister in writing are more of a social than of a moral nature. You might make this address from the pulpit on some early significant occasion having alerted the press, as is your wont. Better still, you could arrange for all the Bishops to give forth simultaneously – una voce so to speak – of a Sunday morning. Indeed a number of your Episcopal colleagues, who have no objection to the scheme, would be delighted by this opportunity to clear the air. I know that you have the authority to pull rank on any who would dissent from this approach. If you draw the line even the Bishop of Galway will toe it.

While I do not wish to be overly prescriptive, the tenor of your address might go something like this.

The Hierarchy wishes to dispel rumours which have been abroad regarding their position on the Government's proposed Mother and Child Scheme. Recognising its duty to give guidance to its followers, the Church has examined the proposal in detail. It is true that, at the beginning, certain members of the Hierarchy wished to seek other opinion before giving the scheme their imprimatur. This seeking of opinion is commonplace in medicine, in the law, in politics and so it is also in theology. It brings the advantage of collective wisdom. The Church considers that it rightly has a role in guiding society and is decidedly of the view that the Government should encourage self-reliance rather than dependency in the citizens. It is nevertheless conceded that, in the interests of social justice, State intervention is necessary in certain areas particularly healthcare. The appalling level of maternal and child mortality in Ireland makes this a suitable case for such State intervention and the Bishops applaud the Minister for his efforts in this regard. We find no theological objection to his scheme. Guided by the Gospel of St Matthew we have reached the conclusion that the physical health of the people is rightly the business of government while their spiritual welfare is the business of the Church.

I earnestly encourage your Grace and the Hierarchy to issue such a public statement. This step will begin the process of defining the boundaries between Church and State and will fortify both. The vultures are circling to pick both our carcasses. As a politician I see my fate clearly. You however are somewhat isolated from such vulgarity. Be assured however that your enemies exist and that by resisting this legislation you will give them succour. The Bishops may of course, in the short term win the battle but ultimately they will most assuredly lose the war.

In conclusion, Archbishop, I wish to make my position entirely clear. Notwithstanding my Catholic faith and my regard and affection for you personally, I intend to stand by the Republic and enact this legislation without delay

Yours sincerely

John A. Costello, Taoiseach.

Cometh the hour, however, absent the man. Of all who have held that great office this Taoiseach was the least likely to resist the Hierarchy. In March 1951 he is preparing to sacrifice the Minister for Health to the wishes of the Bishops.

How the doyens of medicine must have been rejoicing. Secure in their fortress hospitals, Bishop ruled but publicly funded, they could now take their foot off the pedal. They knew that their hated Minister had bitten off more than he could chew, and that his quaint adherence to principle rather than pragmatism, would prevent him from turning. The Minister would be consigned to history and, equally important, the stuffing would be knocked out of his Department of Health mandarins for a generation.

16

MEDICS AND MANDARINS

The relationship between medicine and civil service mandarins was, and remains, enigmatic and fraught. The mandarins viewed the doctors with suspicion and this suspicion was reciprocated and leavened with no small measure of condescension. This hauteur was entirely without justification, since the intellectual calibre of the civil service cadre then, as judged by entry requirements, was vastly superior to that of many doctors who only had to stump up a few quid and present themselves for the pre-medical course.

A STRONG FARMER

The social norms of the time, particularly in so far as they applied to medicine and Church, might well be exemplified by the predicament of a strong farmer with three sons. Ignoring the principle of primogeniture, the least promising academically would be 'kept at home' to work and inherit the land.

The ablest academically would be groomed for the Church. He would proceed to Maynooth where entry requirements to the seminary demanded extremely strong academic grades. There he would be conditioned in the ways of conservatism and piety, the former to the satisfaction of his father, the latter to the delight of his mother. There he would be measured by his academic accomplishments, represented to a significant degree by his mastery of dead languages. Academic advance was matched by intellectual retreat. In the manner of the twenty-first century madrassas of Pakistan, although intelligent, he became de-intellectualised. Any neuronal connections which might have led him to question the received wisdom or the prevailing social order, gradually atrophied and he became a stout defender of the *status quo*.

Our strong farmer of three sons has still to get another off the land and towards this end he often turned to the professions. Historically it was considered, rather pompously, that there were, apart from the oldest of all, only three true professions, the Church, the law and medicine. It would not be in the nature of such a man to put too many eggs in one basket. Furthermore, the countryman does not have much truck with the law and is wary of its denizens: he feels that they keep a closed shop. By contrast he and his wife are well familiar with the local family doctor and would mightily aspire to such a position for their son, as captured in undergraduate doggerel of the time.

> With stethoscope and big top hat
> Mrs McGrath wouldn't you like that

Notwithstanding the student wag who might regale his colleagues late of an evening with such doggerel, the truth is that the intake to medical schools was, in general, academically inferior to that of the Junior Executive Officers joining the civil service at that time. Indeed, many a strong farmer, having the right material, did steer his son in this latter direction.

THE FIFTY POUND MAN

Let us consider then the career progress of two young men. The first is academically strong and is creamed off the top for the civil service. The other, perhaps indeed from the same school or parish, is academically stolid if not a plodder. In those days, before the Central Applications Office (CAO) introduced an element of democracy into these procedures, this latter one, in order to enter medical school, merely had to pony up the fee.

From the day they leave school these two boys, one significantly more gifted than the other, are on widely divergent courses.

The junior civil servant is immediately, by the standards of the time, on the pig's back. He is, in the verbiage of impecunious times, 'earning'. His less endowed counterpart, for whose academic accomplishments he probably had some measure of disdain, drops completely off his radar. The neophyte civil servant is living in the present with his newly found, albeit modest, income, his independence and his significant, albeit again modest, status. At the age of eighteen he has achieved the coveted, if somewhat stultifying, status of being 'permanent and pensionable'. His parents furthermore, in the era of large families, are delighted to have him off their books.

Meanwhile the lesser of our two academic heroes, who disappeared into the medical school, continues to be a burden on his parents and is always strapped for cash. The occasional total dunderhead is weeded out early, and probably never gets past pre-med. The remainder are of sufficient accomplishment to negotiate the examinations and advance steadily through the interminable years of medical undergraduate life. Those interminable years are rather easy-going and would not, in those days, be described as academically frantic. Indeed, elements of the humanities, commerce, engineering and other faculties often mocked the dilatory progress of their medical fellow students. They missed the point however. The long medical course afforded time for mental development and maturation, particularly in male students many of whom, in those half-starved days, were scarcely beyond puberty when they went up to university. A further factor in this maturation, lacking in the modern epoch, was the daily exposure of medical students to their senior professors – indeed the very doyens of medicine of whom, in other respects, we are being censorious.

The effects of this leisurely maturation and role modelling were good and bad.

On the positive side latent talent was, from unpromising beginnings, allowed to develop, indeed on occasions achieving distinction. The downside however was more subtle. The less endowed student began to take on the affect, attitudes and expectations of his role models, the doyens. In short, he developed a sense of entitlement out of proportion to his talents. This cult of entitlement has bedevilled all elites in Ireland, Church, political and professional alike, and always to the detriment of the citizen.

It was this cult of entitlement embedded in his medical adversaries that Dr Noël Browne, Minister for Health, now faced in 1950 and it would bring him down.

Many years pass and our two heroes, now less youthful, make their separate and divergent ways in life.

The civil servant progresses steadily to positions of responsibility and power. His virtues are his lack of flamboyance and his loyalty to and respect for elected politicians. His intellect, although somewhat blunted by years of bureaucratic toil, enables him to have a realistic appraisal of his entitlement. His monetary rewards are solid if not spectacular, and any relative deficiency is more than compensated for by his access to that intangible currency – power.

Contemporaneously our doctor has been making his way in practice and, an industrious worker, he is beginning to prosper. He is not weighed down by the kind of intellectual machinery which would cause him to feel fortunate: instead, he carries a great burden of entitlement. He feels himself to be – long before twenty-first century peddlers of cosmetics distilled the concept – 'worth it'. Stereotypically, he involves himself in medical politics and is a stalwart of the doctor's trade union. It is a feature of all trade unions, particularly those of doctors and lawyers, that they will abandon all rational thought and reason, and argue, even in the face of the most incontrovertible evidence, for the preservation of their powers and privileges – they carry their burden of entitlement with conviction.

Our prosperous doctor, perhaps the lesser of our two heroes, makes an excellent mouthpiece for the more accomplished puppeteer doyens of medicine who in 1950 – *noblesse oblige* after all – did not wish to compromise their dignity by resort to the bull horn. He is a metaphor for the body of the profession. The attributes of being educated, articulate and urbane makes him a formidable adversary in negotiations. He believes in his cause and argues with the utmost conviction. Even against the most incontrovertible evidence, well presented, he believes in the rectitude of his case. Quite simply, he is 'worth it'.

CAVEAT

Towards countering the arguments of those who may not agree with the analysis being presented here several caveats may be entered.

Firstly, those who rise to the top of medicine, as distinct from those who make lots of money out of it, are usually very accomplished scientifically and academically. It is readily conceded that, in 1950, there were many such amongst those whom we are calling the doyens. Indeed their adroit orchestration of events lends support to this view. They knew that, while they needed their megaphone men, one whisper in the ear of the Archbishop of Dublin was worth more than all the shouting.

Secondly, since the time under discussion, the demographic of medicine has changed completely. The days of our stereotype presenting himself to the Bursar at University College Cork with fifty quid are long gone. Entry now, although biased against males because of their later maturation, as mentioned earlier, is mainly by measurement. Entry to medical school is now perceived as fairer and credit for this should be given to politics rather than to the medical establishment. It remains moot, however, whether the incubated entrants to today's medical schools, while costing them a great deal more to produce, will be of any more value to the taxpayers than their more spontaneous antecedents of yesteryear. Indeed, while conceding that it hardly amounts to evidence, many a professor will opine that his worst undergraduate nightmare, on occasion, morphed into the most valuable of practitioners.

The third point of caution emerges from the second above. It is unfair to stigmatise the medical faculty alone as having been peopled by 'fifty pound men'. With the exception of the engineering faculty – where accomplishment in higher mathematics was required – the only requirement for entry to most faculties was ability to pay the fee. Nevertheless it is not comfortable for a medical observer to compare the infrastructural contribution of his own profession to that of the engineers who, at that very time, were bringing a flow of electrons in the form of rural electrification to every remote part of Ireland. And all of this was done by engineers in the type of salaried public employment so detested by the Irish Medical Association.

Minister for Health Noël Browne was intent on doing for medicine (or at least for obstetrical medicine) what the engineers were doing for light: he would make it available to everybody regardless of rank or station. He was, however, up against sterner stuff than a farmer who saw little advantage to himself in the planting of a pylon in the middle of his fine field. The doyens of medicine, and their patsy the Archbishop of Dublin, would see to it that no alien pylon was planted in the middle of their patch. Some will argue, and perhaps not entirely without justification, that the challenges of providing healthcare greatly exceeded those of providing electricity. This, however, was before the appearance of today's advanced medical technology. Indeed the technology of electrification, at that time, was more complex than that required for safe obstetrical practice. Naysayers should ponder whether it was the leaders of

Engineering or Medicine in 1950 who better discharged their respective responsibility to the future infrastructure of the nation.

Our two heroes, the greater and the lesser academically, exemplify the tensions in the relationship between mandarins and medicine. For many years on diverging courses these two personalities, honed by their respective working environments and cultures, are now on a converging path as the civil servant, representing the Department of Health, and his long lost acquaintance meet across the negotiating table. The encounter is not likely to result in happiness.

The mandarin is taken aback to encounter his forgotten acquaintance of yesteryear in such a strong position. To his further discomfiture his adversary is comporting himself with an unexpected self-assurance and urbanity. The civil servant, by his ability and training, is an accomplished dissimulator, and is conditioned not to betray his personal feelings. Nevertheless, he has to summon all his reserves of professionalism to conceal his visceral condescension towards his intellectual inferior of yesteryear, now ensconced across the negotiating table. He has to resist the mistake of thinking that the clock stopped away back then when he was king of the academic castle.

Our lesser hero, by contrast, has been looking forward to the encounter with his illustrious erstwhile acquaintance, the senior Department of Health official, who is much mentioned and little loved in the gossipy dispatches which permeate the medical world. He is possessed of that self-assurance which the competent but not brilliant begin to exhibit to excess when they make money. To the discomfiture of his adversary, he is able to deploy in abundance those props which are emblematic of material success. He motors in style and while not perhaps a fop, he is expensively sartorially elegant. In short, he is inclined to lapse into the kind of ostentation that the sound mandarin despises and eschews. In contrast, those sound public servants of 1950, and for many years thereafter, were perceived as somewhat heroic. For the most part the asceticism which they affected was due to virtue rather than lack of opportunity although, a cynic might observe, the former is much easier in the presence of the latter. Certainly their modern day successors are less cursed by asceticism. Grade inflation and grandiosity of titles (e.g. Secretary General as distinct from the traditional title of Secretary of a Department) enables them to separate the taxpayer from an altogether larger amount of his money.

These two gentlemen are a metaphor for the eternal tension which exists between Ministers for Health and their officers, and the beast that is the organised medical profession.

The conditioning of the worthy civil servant is towards the protection of the public purse against all comers, not least amongst whom is the medical profession when in full negotiating mode. As the State advanced into medicine in the twentieth century, they became extremely restless bedfellows. The mandarin, on occasion, found his conditioning stretched to the full asking himself the question, why must I deal with this tiresome fellow of dubious intellect who clearly has sectional rather than national interest at heart? He is decidedly of the view that the negotiating doctor and all his tribe are not 'worth it.'

The lesser of our two metaphoric heroes, who represents medicine, brings to the relationship an entirely different mindset. His mission is the polar opposite to that of the negotiating civil servant: he must, on behalf of himself and his associates, extract the maximum amount possible from the public purse. He must, in addition, as in his resistance to the Mother and Child Scheme and many others, fight for the preservation of private medical practice. Two purses, after all, are better than one.

A New Minister

It is likely that history in these matters will look with more favour on the mandarin than the medic. The former however, although sometimes dubbed the permanent Government, has much to put up with. While an incumbent Taoiseach might naturally tend to appoint a doctor as Minister for Health, it is generally not the stars of the medical firmament who resort to politics.

Ministers for Health, be they doctors or otherwise, generally fall into two types.

The first is a fellow whose ambitions are consummated by his arrival in the Minister's chair. He is a loyal party supporter who has served his time and proposes to act as a comfortable caretaker. He will abide by the wishes of his party leader and will be guided by his departmental officials. He will do neither good nor harm. The mandarins would wish that all Ministers were thus and that the permanent Government could get on with the business of running the department. Under him the Department of Health is a house of harmony: the proper people are in charge. Such a Minister makes little demands of the Department of Finance. He gives the Taoiseach no trouble – contrast this to Noël Browne in 1950 – and he does not engage in tedious advocacy for his Department. He survives heaves and reshuffles and his endurance in ministerial office is in direct proportion to his ineffectuality.

The second fellow is an entirely different proposition.

He arrives like Christ come to cleanse the Temple.

His coming may have been well trumpeted by the press and the opinion polls. While denizens of the Department tend to take campaign rhetoric with a pinch of salt, there is nevertheless a gathering consternation at the unpredictability, unaffordability and the grandiosity of his un-costed proposals. At this point it seems fair to continue to discourse in the masculine, since all but one of the Ministers for Health have been male and, in any case, the female exception lacked nothing in temple cleansing zeal.

The new Minister then is determined to make his mark. Great populist schemes of global entitlement, divorced from economic reality and with little attention to the tedium of resources, are paraded before a population gorged on expectation. There were, of course, elements of this populism in the Minister's proposed Mother and Child Scheme of 1950. He, however, had embarked upon an incremental, carefully costed and fully funded programme which foundered not upon the rock of finance but upon that of Episcopal objection. There was nothing grandiose about the scheme.

When a zealous and grandiose Minister for Health arrives in the Department, particularly in straitened economic times, his officials make a show of accommodating his follies and foibles while at the same time embarking upon a policy of containment. While the loyalty and discretion of civil servants is much to be admired, occasional vignettes about their antics leak into the medical grapevine.

Mandarins hate nothing more than a loose cannon Minister who announces big bang schemes of reform oblivious of the need for money to implement them. Token schemes, which cost little and can be launched with much fanfare, can be useful in distracting such a Minister and deceiving him into believing that he is leaving his mark.

'The Patient's Charter' of 1992 was a classic example of one such distraction. Nailed to every hospital door of a Monday morning it was supposed – if we may presume upon Martin Luther again – to 'reform' the health service. Its utopian aims, plagiarised from the British National Health Service, where it was of course properly funded, filled the bloated news media for weeks. In this regard the mandarins have a slavish admiration for the British Health Service in which few of them, as distinct from doctors and nurses, have ever worked. They have refined a most tiresome methodology of waiting until some new British measure has begun to fail before discovering it and introducing it to Ireland.

MEDICAL PARADOX

The uneasy interface between medic and mandarin exhibits an interesting paradox.

It is the duty of doctors, and many have answered that call, to advocate on behalf of patients for better medical services. At the same time it is the duty of doctors' trade unions (often referred to as professional organisations, the word 'union' being anathema to the more urbane end of society) to extract the maximum possible rewards on behalf of their members – this is fair enough. Or is it?

Extracting maximum rewards for the doctors can impact negatively on the patient in two ways. Firstly, and more simply, it depletes the pot of money available for the provision of services. Secondly, it can, and on many occasions does, cause the profession to resist the implementation of policies, structures and programmes which would be in the interest of patients, but perceived not to be in the material interest of doctors. This latter effect is destructive out of all proportion to the previous and, in a country of pork barrel politics, has bedevilled the Irish Health Service. The population understands the first – the money. It does not understand the second – the importance of structure – and has been vulnerable to spurious argument and, in the case of the Mother and Child Scheme, to outright deception.

It is easier to deceive the public if first you succeed in deceiving yourself. Thus, a doctor could indulge himself in the schizoid luxury of piously declaiming his support for the patient's every need, while at the same time instructing his organisation to oppose and frustrate the development of structures which would fulfil that need. He could have his cake and eat it.

17

THE MEMORANDUM

It is likely that the Minister for Health knows at this time that his Mother and Child Scheme is a dead duck and his political career an extremely lame one. He is not writing therefore with any hope of resuscitating his project. Rather his purpose is to enter the shameful facts into the official record: he is writing for history. But he will not wait for history. He is preparing, the moment he goes down, to flout all convention, and send the entire sorry correspondence to the press. If he is to be damned, he may as well publish and be damned.

The arguments presented in the 'Ferns' letter, the Minister concedes agreeably, 'are of such importance that he feels it is necessary for him to reply at some length'. If one might paraphrase his thoughts at this time, and if his decorum had slipped, this latter sentence might have read, 'the arguments presented on behalf of the Hierarchy are so fatuous and devoid of substance, that I can easily demolish them with reasoned argument and I will now proceed to do so publicly and at some length'.

The Minister opens his rebuttal of Their Lordships' position by reiterating that the scheme will be voluntary, comparing it to primary education.

> Every parent will be free to avail of it or not ... just as state-aided primary schools are provided for such as wish to attend them.

The Minister suggests, with some condescension, that Their Lordships have failed to grasp the essence of the matter: they are suffering from a 'misapprehension'. His endeavour to help them out of their confusion by comparing his scheme to the schools lacked validity.

The primary schools were on Catholic autopilot, with the local parish priest controlling and having the power of life and death over the State-paid teachers. The parish priest, indeed usually a benign manager, had rarely to rouse himself: the compliance of the teachers preserved the tranquillity of his, often pastoral, existence.

Under this regime the priority was religious instruction, often to the detriment of reading, writing and arithmetic. Indeed, as confirmation time approached, and as an inspection by His local Lordship beckoned, the three Rs were sometimes suspended completely. Thus would the teacher bask in the reflected glory of the piety instilled into her pupils. Under this regime very few teachers bucked the traces by deviating from Catholic orthodoxy, and the occasional miscreant was dealt with in summary fashion.

The Archbishop knew full well that he had an iron grip on the schools and, with the publicly funded teacher training colleges sporting profoundly Catholic names, that would endure. A lazy theocratic State was happy to leave that and much else to the Church. While the Church held the power, the State paid but retained vicarious responsibility – these vicarious chickens would eventually come home to roost to the taxpayer in many expensive guises.

Unlike in the schools, however, the Archbishop of Dublin and the Hierarchy generally saw their hegemony in their flagship hospitals threatened. That such institutions, with their affectation of moral (and indeed scientific) superiority, were about to be invaded by un-Irish activities was something up with which His Grace of Dublin would not put. The maestro in Drumcondra was confident that, with one twitch of his baton, the State would be turned away from the evils of 'State medicine' and its citizens would continue to enjoy, or endure, the standards of those Southern European countries where prelates, like him, cohabiting with politicians of the right, held sway.

> The only fundamental difference in principle between the existing Public Assistance system of medical relief and the proposed Mother and Child Service is that there was a means test for the former and that it will be eliminated for the latter.

> The Minister presumes that the elimination of the means test could not be a factor which weighed with the Hierarchy in arriving at the opinion quoted above.

The forensic logic of the Minister's argument, placed before a jury, would have carried the day hands down. He was not however to be judged by a jury of his peers but rather by a secret conclave, itself under the malign spell of his nemesis McQuaid.

The Minister for Health states, correctly, that his proposed measures are no more than a further quantitative increment of a long established medico-social trend: a trend to which Their Lordships had never objected before (i.e., before the Health Act of 1947). They must therefore, he assumes, be objecting to some new ingredient. The only new ingredient, or 'fundamental difference in principle', was, of course, the absence of a means test. The argument proceeds with a logic worthy of Euclid. If you are in favour of a means test, it follows that you are against motherhood and apple pie.

Then the Minister proceeds to taunt the Hierarchy. His tone is somewhat evocative of John McEnroe's outburst to the tennis umpire: 'you can not be serious'.[141] How could they possibly object, in the face of such incontrovertible logic, to a much needed compassionate scheme in which, up to now,

Their Lordships had been unable to point out any moral flaw? Furthermore, he had compromised on the clauses to which they had objected and even agreed that they, the Bishops, submit their own modification of those clauses for inclusion. Then with derision he gives the Hierarchy the benefit of the doubt. He assumes, with mock credulity, that they are not sufficiently daft as to find the absence of a means test in some mysterious way, contrary to the law of God. Such a position would be so outlandish that he assumes 'the elimination of the mean test could not be a factor' in causing them to object to his scheme.

The Minister for Health is proposing 'better and more extensive hospital treatment facilities'. Surely the disciples of Hippocrates must embrace this prospect with enthusiasm. Well, as Sir Humphrey Appleby[142] would say, yes and no.

Yes, there were doctors in favour of the Minister's proposal. These would be a subset that, in the best tradition, would always support and work towards the improvement of facilities, services and structures. Even amongst this modest number however, the Minister's support would be thinned out by an unwillingness to take a stand against the known position of their Church.

The naysayers would fall into two groups.

The first group, feeling financially threatened but at least admirable for their honesty, would say, 'Hippocrates be damned, we need to make a living'.

The second element, fearing loss of income and control, would find it more convenient to surrender to the comfort of the spurious moral argument promulgated on their behalf by no less an authority than the Bishops. Their argument, of admirable simplicity but spectacular vacuity was, 'the Bishops are against it, it must be wrong'.

The Minister continues his memorandum to the Bishops with sweet reasonableness:

> The letter from the Hierarchy goes on to state that the right to provide for the health of children belongs to parents. The Minister, naturally, is in complete agreement with this view.

The Hierarchy wrote with bizarre obliquity of 'the right of parents', rather than as most people would see it, the duty, to provide for the health of their children. The Minister, indeed agreeably, points out that he also is against any invasion of parental rights. Implicit in his argument, however, is the idea that a right, without the material means to exercise it, is no right at all. Indeed under the prevailing socio-medical regime the rights of many parents and children, while theoretically abundant, were in reality extremely skeletal. The Minister for Health was now proposing to put meat on those bones.

Those diminishing few who remember urban and rural Ireland of 1950 might indeed wonder with puzzlement which rights were threatened. Seeing little evidence of such rights, particularly when compared to healthcare available in the civilised world generally, a poor person, or indeed one not so poor, might wonder why Their Lordships were so exercised. The Minister was not proposing to deprive parents of any right: he proposed rather to provide them with the means to exercise the right to 'provide for the health of their children' – this quotation taken verbatim from the Bishop of Ferns' letter. Noël Browne is adroitly showing that the Bishops are arguing against themselves. In 1950 it was not the Minister for Health who was invading the family but rather the clergy who amounted to a third, almost voyeuristic, presence in every marital bedroom. In front of a jury the Bishops' case would flop and peals of derision would echo from the public gallery. He presiding over the packed jury at Maynooth, however, would reach for the black cap.

The Minister's next passage on 'education' exposes the narrow Irish vernacular definition of morality in 1950.

> The aspects which have moral implications will continue under the new scheme to be in the care of the family, or the members of the medical profession who have care of them at present.

'Moral implications' as used here means the Ferns taboo triad of 'sex relations, chastity and marriage'. Indeed the Minister for Health falls prey to this thinking. Matters that have 'moral implications' are hived off by him for special consideration: these are the business of Bishops. Markers of poverty, several of which the Minister mentions, for example appalling dental and personal hygiene and the means to correct them, which apparently lack a moral dimension, are in an entirely separate category. Such deprivation and all its accompaniments were areas, according to the Minister for Health, 'into which moral issues do not enter' – morality as so defined did not encompass social morality. Referring to such social matters the Minister states clearly:

> It is only the latter type of education which is to be provided under the scheme.

Then Noël Browne offers complete surrender by stating that he was:

> ... prepared to submit to the Hierarchy for their approval the draft, when available, of that part of the regulations which will deal with these matters.

The Minister now, having agreed to 'meet the requirements of the Hierarchy', is in full retreat. Gone is the feistiness which has heretofore sustained him. Gone is the rhetoric of 'none may refute'. The Archbishop has trimmed the hair of Samson and all his power is draining away. Now, too late, in the theocratic Ireland of 1950, he knows who may and who may not 'refute'. How excruciating it must have been for him to compose the statement 'the Minister is prepared to submit to the Hierarchy'.

Indeed it is not comfortable to read his pleading even at a remove of more than six decades, when the *dramatis personae, pro and contra*, are long departed.

At no stage in the lengthy saga did the Hierarchy make a constructive proposal to the Minister. The Minister now, perhaps with some irony, is giving them the opportunity to do so. He is 'prepared to consider' any suggestions they might make to break the impasse. The Archbishop, however, now fully in control of a sycophantic Taoiseach and a supine cabinet, has no intention of engaging in constructive dialogue with the despised and soon to be abandoned upstart Minister. When the hounds smell blood they do not back off – and so it is also with the hounds of God.

The Minister, in his memorandum, now proceeds to try to reassure the Bishops on the matter of 'gynaecological care' and 'medical advice' under the proposed scheme. Fundamental to that care are the medical personnel who would be administering it, and the Bishops' anxiety that they might have been trained in institutions in which the Hierarchy had 'no confidence'. With regard to making such medical appointments the Minister cites Article 44 of the constitution as prohibiting 'any discrimination on the grounds of religious profession'.

It speaks volumes of the relationship between Church and State that the Minister for Health, by way of justifying his actions, must, defensively, point out to the religious leadership the legal process governing 'the recruitment of medical personnel' to the public service. The proposed Mother and Child Scheme envisaged a much expanded role for family doctors in the provision of such services.

Family practice in Ireland in 1950 was poorly developed and there was altogether more emphasis on, and prestige attached to, hospital rather than community medicine. This imbalance, ideal for neither medicine nor the community, suited the Hierarchy sitting as they were astride the major leadership hospitals. The Minister's proposal, while it contained much about hospitals, would nudge the equilibrium away from them. Also, the family doctor, as the first point of contact with the system, was the most likely to give advice – about birth control. This worried the Hierarchy that their control of Irish medicine would begin to drag its anchor.

Another factor was that during the Second World War, and its economically depressed aftermath, there were few career opportunities for doctors in Ireland. The diminished output of the medical schools was largely for export, for the most part to England where many Irish doctors found employment in the National Health Service and a lesser number, as had been traditional,[143] in the armed forces.

It has been a historical feature of the Irish health service that whenever there is expansion, the medical diaspora apply, in considerable numbers, for the new posts. Such 'wild geese' doctors were, and still tend to be, of greater accomplishment and broader vision than their stay at home colleagues who spared themselves the rigours of such travel and the mind broadening influence of alternative systems – educational, scientific and social.

Mind-broadened medical elements returning from England, to take up posts in which they would have a role in the education of women in 'sex relations chastity and marriage', was certainly enough to stress the digestion of the Archbishop of Dublin beyond its limited tolerance of things Anglo Saxon.

The Minister's next gambit does credit neither to himself nor to the medical profession.

> There is an additional safeguard that, unlike the neighbouring island, this country is predominantly Catholic and its medical profession is predominantly Catholic also.

He makes much of the fact that the medical community in Ireland, as distinct from that of what he rather strangely calls the neighbouring island (don't mention England), 'is predominantly Catholic'. The fact that most doctors in Ireland were Catholics should have been neither here nor there but the Minister, with naïveté, uses it as a crutch. The Hierarchy could, in the last analysis he points out, rely on the medical profession to do their bidding and enforce their diktats. This was probably as true as it was unflattering. It is indeed probable that many doctors, in so far as they thought about it at all, rather like the Taoiseach, considered themselves first Catholics and second doctors – Catholic doctors rather than doctor Catholics. As long as the Hierarchy remained in the ascendant many, devoid of ideology, would go with the flow.

In many instances this posture would have been determined by pragmatic economic factors rather than ideology. There existed, however, doctors who were Catholic ideologues of sincere conviction, and who were unyielding in their determination to promote, or indeed enforce, Catholic orthodoxy on the practice of medicine in general.

An example of such a movement – emblematic of the time – was 'the Irish Guild of St Luke SS Cosmas and Damien,[144] a society of Catholic doctors which existed in Ireland since Blueshirt times (1934). This might be characterised as a self-styled Catholic medical moral militia. Predictably, minutes of meetings have excessive resort to use of the word 'moral' to which they seemed to accord themselves proprietorial rights. Equally predictable was the obsession with contraception, abortion and all matters related to the dreaded matter of sex. Obstetrician gynaecologists, who were deemed sound on these topics, were invited speakers at meetings. Presidents of Catholic seminary schools were invited to give a disquisition of their unsurprising views on such matters.[145] While the prime movers in such a medical group might today be regarded as having been something of a fringe, perusal of their minutes leads to a different assessment: a great many prominent doctors, particularly obstetrician gynaecologists, and other academics, participated in one way or another.

This then was the atmosphere in which the Minister for Health, to the dismay of such independent medical thinkers as may have existed, and to his own discredit, took it upon himself to reassure the Hierarchy that the 'predominantly Catholic' medical profession could be used as a reliable tool to enforce their policies.

Turning to the bogus issue of medical confidentiality, already dealt with in Chapter 5, the Minister states, 'The Mother and Child Scheme will not introduce any new principle in this regard.'

Medical Confidentiality Syndrome, if we may so call it, is typically unleashed when, as in this instance of 1950, the Department of Health attempts to introduce some new measure which is perceived detrimental to doctor's finances or liberties. When schemes are well funded and the doctors are happy, as in the General Medical Services Scheme (1972) – which represented perhaps the greatest invasion of medicine by the State up to that time – medical confidentiality was not an issue.

Doctors protest about medical confidentiality when it suits their purpose and do not always defend it when they should. Such an example, fresh in the mind at the time of writing, is the process by which United States intelligence services abused a poliomyelitis vaccination programme in Pakistan in order to confirm, by the DNA of his children, and the reprehensible abuse of his sister's medical records in the USA, the identity of Osama Bin Laden in order to set up his extra-judicial killing. The consequence of this was the loss of credibility of the vaccination programme, and the murder of several of its operatives – Osama is dead but polio lives in Pakistan.[146]

While it is alarming that a constitutional democracy resorts to such an abuse of medical records, what is most remarkable is the lack of outrage from medical leaders and from the captive news media to this abuse of privileged medical access. When, however, doctors feel threatened about their conditions, meetings which normally struggle to achieve a quorum have standing room only. The bleachers are crowded with non-season ticket holders and up goes the shout of medical confidentiality.

Noël Browne eviscerates Their Lordships' argument with the simple statement:

> The Minister feels that the doctor patient relationship would not be impaired under the scheme.

So contrarian is the position of the Hierarchy that the Minister for Health, in his memorandum to them, appears to feel the need to defend the very existence of medical records. He points out that all hospitals, including presumably those presided over by Bishops and Archbishops, must maintain medical records. He is suggesting that medical records in 'the local authority service' are no less secure than those held privately. The medical profession's record in Ireland in the area of confidentiality has been excellent and did not need shoring up by intervention of the Hierarchy.

PRIVATE AND PRIVATE

The 'elimination' of private medical practice is as undesirable as it is impossible.

> ... the Minister submits that the scheme will not result in the elimination of private medical practitioners.

All medical encounters should be, and are, private in the true sense of the word. The word private, as used thus, refers to the intimate personal clinical detail discussed between doctor and patient – this is sacrosanct.

The word private takes on an entirely different meaning, however, when it is applied to administrative structures governing the provision of medical services. Here the word refers to the means by which the service is paid for – it has nothing whatever to do with medical confidentiality. The matter of whether the service is paid for by the patient herself, or by the public purse, has nothing to do with the protection of intimate medical detail, and it was the height of mischief for the Hierarchy to suggest otherwise.

Those funded by the public purse are often referred to by the demeaning and unprofessional misnomer as 'public patients'. Those paying for their treatment themselves are referred to by the more flattering, if not always more reassuring, title as 'private patients'. There are thus two kinds of privacy – privacy of payment and privacy of intimate medical details. The flaw in the Bishops' argument was they posited that you could not have the latter without the former. This flawed analysis was unsupported by evidence, erosive of patients' trust in confidentiality, profoundly unflattering to doctors and the public service generally, and reflective of an extremely pessimistic view of human nature.

A rare point of agreement between this writer and the Hierarchy of 1950, albeit for different reasons, is that the 'elimination of private medical practitioners', then as now, would have been extremely undesirable. Competition is the essence of all functioning systems and without it there is a slide into mediocrity or worse. The abolition of private medicine, or its 'elimination', in the words of the Bishop of Ferns, would be a disaster for standards in Ireland. It was not, indeed, that the Archbishop of Dublin was a doctrinaire advocate of competition; quite the reverse was the case. He was insecure about the competition of a small rump of Protestants. There was little doubt that he would, if it had been within his power, have wiped *The Irish Times* from the face of the earth. And, most of all, he was less than sanguine regarding the competition which Noël Browne's proposals presaged for his bastion hospitals.

While private medicine is in itself no bad thing, it is not necessarily the case that if some is good, more is better and most is best. At the time of writing builders and developers, having turned the economy of Ireland into a disaster area, seek to morph their empty shells into hospitals. In so doing it is likely that they will achieve for medical standards what they did for the national economy. One is minded of the surfeit of television channels with few worth watching and ironically perhaps the best of those, publicly funded.

'Private medical practitioners', that species of which the Hierarchy were so solicitous, will always exist. Even if the Minister for Health had wished to kill them off, he would have been wasting his efforts. Private medical practice is like a bacterium, and paternalistic governments have, time and again, tried to kill it off with huge doses of socialism. Repeated heavy doses of Government largesse, it is true, attenuate its vigour for a time, but gradually it marshals its defences in the knowledge that its day will come again when the spendthrift and profligate politicians have emptied the national coffers.

Private medicine did not need the Archbishop of Dublin or the massed ranks of the Hierarchy to defend it. It is more ancient and visceral than that. Like the tuberculous disease found in ancient Egyptian mummies it simply hangs around to await more opportune times. The large doses of streptomycin which the Minister for Health was lavishing on the tubercle bacillus would not wipe it out but would rather result in the emergence of a more virulent strain. So it is also when the Government applies large doses of socialism to health; the organism of private practice, vulnerable to the toxin of Government largesse, becomes dormant. It always re-emerges, however, mutated, leaner and better adapted to its environment than before.

There have been times and places where the enemies of private medicine succeeded in making it scarcely respectable. Such endeavours are usually full of hypocrisy. In the workers' paradise of Lenin the insiders, although depriving the masses of choice, maintained private medical facilities for themselves. In Britain's free for all National Health Service, private practice took a big hit. It became *démodé* for luminaries to 'go private'. It became more than his life was worth – his political life that is – for a politician to seek his medical salvation in a private institution. But as Britain's coffers emptied, denuded by daft wars, populist largesse and the evaporation of imperial booty, 'going private' regained its cachet. Private medicine, resistant to all the ideological poisons, is back.

But it was about Ireland that the Hierarchy were worried in 1950. Other countries in Northern Europe, in their development of public health services, allowed the private side to equilibrate at a new much lower level. The Archbishop of Dublin however, was a believer in big Church rather than big Government and therefore advocated the contrary position. The language used by the Hierarchy is pejorative towards public medicine – the Minister's Mother and Child Scheme was, according to the Bishop of Ferns, 'a costly bureaucratic scheme of nationalised medical service'. It was the public, not the private element of health provision, which the Hierarchy wished to equilibrate at a lower level.

The Archbishop of Dublin would sublimate the welfare of his followers to his fanatical desire to keep the State out of medicine. He did not know that you cannot keep the State, at least one which is worth the name, out of medicine. Events in America, citadel of capitalism, provide proof, if proof be needed, with the arrival of Government-enforced 'Obamacare'.

The Minister sees a need to reassure the Bishops about private medical practice stating:

> ... he was prepared to give all private medical practitioners an opportunity to participate in the scheme.

> This should remove any possible objection on the ground that the scheme might tend to reduce the amount of traditional private medical practice.

The Minister for Health, in his memorandum, is not writing to doctors reassuring them that their private practice is safe; incomprehensibly, he is offering this reassurance to Bishops.

Ironically, the medical profession has usually benefited materially when the Government brings new and better services to the people, and has benefited psychologically from the emotional dividend of being able to discharge the functions for which it is trained.[147] This, however, was a tough message for the Minister to sell in 1950. Those afflicted by 'lack of means' or 'ignorance' – the huddled masses – would have to wait until the Hierarchy could be rid of this turbulent Minister for Health.

INCONVENIENT STATISTICS

There is more than ample statistical evidence that Ireland, in 1950, was backward with regard to rates of maternal and infant mortality. That a Minister for Health, in his benevolent efforts to address this problem, should be obstructed by Bishops, is today beyond comprehension and is surely indicative that something rotten was afoot. Such, however, was the influence of the Hierarchy on the body politic and the population, that obscurantist non-arguments by the Bishops prevailed over the Minister's sound statistical evidence. Their Lordships exhibited, and got away with, a selective contrived deafness to inconvenient truths – a phenomenon well embedded in the Irish language as *Bodhaire Uí Laoighre*.[148] It is not without significance that the Irish language should provide such a ready-made satirical expression to describe this national tendency towards convenient selective hearing loss. Such was the iron grip of the Church in 1950 that the vast majority of the Catholic population exhibited this affliction.

Referring to 'the high level of mother and child mortality' and the need for 'drastic improvement' in services, Noël Browne goes on to state:

> ... it was the considered view of the Oireachtas in passing
> the Health Act of 1947 that such improvement could
> best be effected by the introduction of a free mother and
> child service.

In Ireland in 1950 the infant mortality rate, as cited by
the Minister in his booklet and extracted from World Health
Organisation statistics, was 41.42 (per 1,000 live births); in the
United States it was 30.46; in Spain it was 63.9. In Sweden, a
country whose mores would certainly not have endeared it to
the prudish Archbishop McQuaid, it was 19.51, less than half
Ireland's rate. Today the United States, with its detestation
of Government health interventions, has fallen behind most
developed countries, as judged by this widely accepted
statistical measurement. The result of Government neglect of
its ghettos, or as the Bishop of Ferns might have put it in 1950,
the avoidance of 'costly bureaucratic scheme[s] of nationalised
medical service', is plain to be seen in the United States which
for many of the intervening years was the richest country in the
world.

On this measure of infant mortality Ireland now ranks
twenty-first in the world in such (almost) acceptable company
as Israel and Australia. The United States, ranked thirty-
fourth, is flanked by Cuba and Malta. Top of the table is a
small new densely populated resource-poor country with the
most interventionist of Governments – Singapore. The more
laissez faire, resource-rich and contiguous, Malaysia, of which
Singapore was part until 1964, languishes in forty-eighth
position.[149]

The figures for maternal mortality convey the same message
as those for infant mortality discussed above. To its immense
credit, Ireland, where all maternity hospitals are now public,
today ranks sixth in the world alongside Singapore – six
maternal deaths per 100,000 deliveries.[150] The United States,
by contrast, with eight deaths ranks eighteenth. This latter is a

lamentable performance which, while considerably exercising liberal commentators, appears to cause the right wing and the big money no anxiety at all.

These comparisons are made, not primarily to censure the United States, but rather to show what bad company the Irish Catholic Hierarchy kept in 1950. They are made to show how badly the Church was led and how receptive it was to the tendentious protestations of the medical leadership. Socialised medicine, as visiting American luminaries liked to call it with ill-concealed condescension, was un-American – a blasphemy against the God of the market.

In the matter of maternal mortality, however, the market has relegated America to number eighteen in the world.

Finally, having defined the magnitude of the problem, the Minister states that the solution was already incubating when he took office. It is probable, however, that he and his cabinet colleagues were unaware that when the scheme had been proposed by the previous Government in 1947, the Hierarchy had also objected.[151] He is merely acting as midwife responding to a broad consensus. He is sticking it to the Hierarchy saying – everybody is in favour of it but you and the doctors.

EPISCOPAL DECOYS

Throughout the controversy the Hierarchy failed to address the nub of the matter and explain why, in their opinion, the Minister's scheme was morally repugnant. They had an excellent reason for this reticence – the scheme was not in the least morally repugnant and they knew it. They, therefore, preferred to argue not about the substantive issue of why a free for all scheme without a means test was the devil's work, but rather about related decoy issues. In short, they were behaving more like politicians than men of God.

Thus the Bishop of Ferns, in his letter as secretary to the Hierarchy, expounds piously on the virtue of attending to infrastructural deficiencies in the Health Service. This was no more than an uncontroversial matter on which there was universal agreement. He is urging the Minister to build hospitals when, in fact, that is precisely what he had been doing for several years. He is admonishing the Minister to direct his attention to 'facilities which are at present lacking' when, in fact, the Minister has been doing precisely that, with energy and to much acclaim, since taking office three years before. It is as if the Hierarchy scarcely knew what was happening in the Health Service generally and cared little about what was happening outside their own bastion hospitals.

The Minister's rebuttal of their points makes the Bishops look silly.

> The Minister has in fact for the last three years been promoting a very large building programme designed to provide maternity hospitals.

> The various measures which are being taken are within the knowledge of individual members of the Hierarchy in regard to their own areas

Here then we see the Hierarchy urging the Minister to improve services while obstructing him in his efforts to upgrade those in most need of improvement – maternity and child health services.

In a strange perversion of the teaching of Jesus Christ, the Hierarchy's position was that to provide care for the sick free of charge was a Godless vice, and that the road to perdition could only be avoided by charging them for it. One is minded of Christ cleansing the Temple of moneychangers and is tempted to venture that a visit to his house in Ireland was long overdue.

The Minister for Health now proceeds to pour ridicule on the Hierarchy for their detachment, and suggests that they do not know what is going on 'in their own areas'. Rhetorically he asks if his 'very large building programme' has escaped their attention. The reason for this detachment was clear enough, but regrettably only to a few. When needing medical attention themselves their Lordships rarely resorted to the Minister's secular type of hospital where contact with the *profanum vulgus* would have afforded therapeutic insights which might have rendered them less cavalier about the predicaments of the common people. Rather they sought out the comfort and discretion of institutions which they themselves controlled. There they had their own designated quarters known on occasion as 'the Bishop's room', the services of a troupe of nuns, control over senior medical appointments and the reassuring ability to stroll down to 'the parlour' to view their own graven image hanging on the wall in the distinguished company of that of their boss in Rome.

Indulging in such trappings, comforts and isolation were scarcely conducive to the development of insight into the health tribulations of the common people. True, few would deny the senior clergy reasonable comfort, but they were unlikely to find the opportunity to anoint Mary Magdalene[152] in such a place. Yet they sought to control the manner in which health services for the less fortunate developed and to frustrate progress in directions not to their liking.

EPISCOPAL TAX ADVISORS

The Hierarchy had taken it upon themselves to offer advice on taxation policy; not everybody would be of the view that this should be their major priority. The Minister, in his memorandum quotes from the Ferns letter:

> ... the State should give adequate maternity benefits and taxation relief for large families.

Their analysis, as presented by the Bishop of Ferns, was superficial and poorly thought through. They advise the Government to lavish tax relief on those who, effectively, were paying little income tax if any at all. The poor, who predominantly were burdened with large families and had little to tax, would not benefit from this measure. It was those of the middle class with large families, who would benefit most. The Bishops, therefore, find themselves arguing, not for the first time,[153] on behalf of those least in need of relief – the comfortable middle class from which they themselves, for the most part, had come.

On the matter of taxation the Hierarchy are now functioning, *par excellence*, in political mode. Their introduction of taxation was a classical political ploy, a decoy, a red herring. They were prepared to introduce any extraneous topic, rather than take on the impossible task of explaining their ludicrous insistence on a means test.

Of all the inventions of the welfare state, precisely the kind of state which John Charles McQuaid was fighting tooth and claw to prevent, nothing is more emblematic than the provision of decent maternity and child health services. There is something of Gilbert and Sullivan about the position into which the Hierarchy had allowed themselves to be painted. The absurdity of demanding more 'maternity benefits' while at the same time insisting that the State should stay out of family matters is worthy of the music hall. But it was no laughing matter. What emerges, yet again, is that the Hierarchy seemed to care little whether or not their argument made sense and were happy to tough it out – sense or no sense. Such was their cavalier abuse of power that they expected the most crass absurdities to pass without demur.

Pounds, Shillings and Pence – and Babies

In his memorandum, the Minister challenges the Hierarchy with evidence that the income tax code is not just enlightened but also family friendly. He is suggesting that the Minister for Finance has little need of Episcopal advice in this regard.

> ... a married man with two children..... pays no income tax unless his income is above the £10. 10s a week level.

A tax-free income of £10.10s in 1950 was reasonable by the standards prevailing in an economically depressed Ireland. Of course this statistic applied only to the 'married man with two children'. This example, either a practitioner of monkish continence or, worse still, improvising some form of contraception, would not particularly have endeared himself to the Archbishop of Dublin; indeed, he fitted more into the Protestant stereotype. One is tempted to observe that the Minister, in citing the example of such an un-Catholic fellow, is doing little for his cause.

The Minister for Health, however, in a master stroke, now resorts to an altogether different stereotype.

> ... a man with eight children pays no income tax unless he has about £16.10s a week.

This commonplace stalwart is altogether more likely to find favour with the Hierarchy. He is precisely of the species which, the Archbishop of Dublin fears, will become extinct if the Minister's intrusion into matters reproductive goes unchecked. The Minister now proceeds to trumpet the support which the State gives to this worthy fellow. He is again telling the Hierarchy that they are either poorly informed or misrepresenting the facts. What they are urging the Government to do has already been done.

This fellow of eight children is the recipient of a tax-free allowance in proportion to his virility and in the happy event of his reaching the apostolic dozen (a far from rare achievement), this tax free allowance would increase to £1,000 per annum – a princely sum indeed in 1950. All of these numbers were a matter of public record and Their Lordships should have trod more carefully. To put these numbers in perspective, the cost of maintaining a boy in one of Their Lordships', admittedly spartan, diocesan secondary boarding schools at the time rarely exceeded £60 per annum.

The State, then, the Minister is pointedly informing the Hierarchy, is demonstrably supportive of the large family in its taxation policy. In addition he is making it clear, to anybody who will do the sums, that further tampering will only steer money to those in least need of it on higher incomes. He is demonstrating to the Bishops that the income tax device which they are suggesting is not suited to their purpose. He is telling them, albeit not in so many words, that their argument is flawed.

The Archbishop of Dublin was, it has emerged, not strong on numbers. When he finally demitted office the Archdioceses of Dublin was broke. The Minister, however, was now spitting out pounds, shillings and pence in rebuttal of the Bishops' misguided foray into matters fiscal.

The Minister goes on to point out yet again that there is no new principle involved in providing supportive services free of any charge:

> ... children's allowances are payable without any means test irrespective of the means of the family if that family contains children within the meaning of the Act.

As an example of the underdeveloped state of social services at the time, the implementation of the 1944 Children's Allowance Act was, enigmatically, the responsibility of the Minister for Industry and Commerce.[154] Also, the Act dealt rather unsympathetically with the less fecund of our earlier two characters, the 'man with two children' – he got nothing. The offspring of this unfortunate fellow were not, in the words of the Act 'qualified children'. The third child and each thereafter qualified for a weekly allowance of two shillings and six pence. The Act, although well intentioned, discriminated against small families and thus favoured Catholics over Protestants. Unsurprisingly, this intrusion of the State into family affairs raised no objection from the Catholic Hierarchy.

MINISTER'S FINAL CHALLENGE

The closing passage of the Minister's memorandum to the Bishops is a gauche combination of conciliation and challenge. He has yielded on everything except the means test. He has capitulated on everything and most particularly on the matter of education for women:

> ... whatever guarantees the Hierarchy desire in the matter of instruction will be unreservedly given.

This is written in order to make the Minister look reasonable when, as is now his intention, he releases the whole sorry correspondence to *The Irish Times*. He knows that the Government will fall and that he is facing an election. He is circumspect that any overt disrespect towards the Hierarchy in that correspondence, regardless of how deserving of such disrespect they might have made themselves, would still damage him in the public eye. But this is more shadow boxing. He is not offering the one guarantee upon which the Bishops are insisting – the imposition of a means test to protect the private practices of their medical cronies.

In addition, for the Minister to offer 'guarantees' to the Hierarchy as to what 'instruction' doctors might offer to women was absurd. He could not possibly regulate such professional interactions and he knew it. Yet again it should be pointed out that 'instruction' was Bishop-speak for the unmentionable business of pregnancy prevention and all the behaviour and paraphernalia pertaining to it. The Archbishop had his own interpretation of what 'instruction' should involve. He would instruct the Government to keep the supply and possession of contraceptives illegal. He would, albeit vicariously, instruct Post Office employees to open people's mail from England and confiscate those rubber goods which were the devil's instruments. And, to its shame, he would instruct a mostly subservient medical profession to enforce Catholic policy in such matters.

The Archbishop of Dublin, John Charles McQuaid, would deal with the matter of 'instruction' himself and he would have no truck with 'guarantees' from the Minister for Health.

Then Noël Browne, rhetorically, offers his final challenge:

> The Minister respectfully asks whether the Hierarchy considers that the Mother and Child Scheme is contrary to Catholic moral teaching.

One last time the Minister taunts Their Lordships: put up or shut up. He is saying to them, ' I know that my Mother and Child Scheme is not "contrary to Catholic moral teaching"; you know that it is not, indeed the dogs in the street know that it is not. Even the doctors, for all their huffing and puffing, know that it is not. You are simply abusing your power.'

Thus ended the Minister's valedictory memorandum – his speech from the dock – which he was not allowed to make.

18

Mindsets

Now that the drama is drawing to a close one might speculate on the respective mindsets of the antagonists, Noël Browne and John Charles McQuaid.

The Minister's Mindset

I am the Minister for Health with my seal of office from the head of State. I am bound by the law of the land, and indeed by the law of God in whom I believe, to provide services for the people to the extent that the economy can sustain. I view this as both my statutory and my Christian duty and am at a loss to find any conflict between the two. I am merely the instrument of the consensus of the duly elected representatives of the Parliament of the people. These latter have found the maternal and infant mortality rates in Ireland to be scandalous and a national disgrace. All political parties are agreed on this. I did not initiate these proposed measures. Indeed I was not in politics when they were conceived. It falls to me now, however, to provide the framework for the implementation of the democratically decreed principles of a Mother and Child Health Service and I propose to do so.

It is normal, Parliament having determined and agreed the 'broad outline' of an Act, for the Minister and his staff, using the instruments described in the Act, to put meat on the bones before the proposed measure is duly voted into law by the House. While I understand the resistance of the medical establishment, I am uncomprehending of the reason why the implementation of this

Act has drawn me into conflict with the Catholic Hierarchy. I have sought enlightenment from them and none has been forthcoming. As an educated Catholic I am familiar with 'Catholic moral teaching.' Furthermore the theological advice which I have sought assures me that in this matter there is no conflict between my Statutory and my Christian duties. If the Bishops will explain to me and to the public the moral basis of their objections to the absence of a free scheme without a means test I will yield, but not before.

The Archbishop of Dublin has captured the levers of power in this State. The Taoiseach and the rest of the cabinet acquiesce in this, I do not. The Archbishop finds my resistance intolerable and a threat to his hegemony. He is abetted by leaders in Medicine whose tendentious arguments sit comfortably with his ideology. His objections are worldly and ideological, not moral.

I am resolved therefore to implement this scheme fully and without a means test, or fall on my sword. If forced so to do, I will inform the people of the facts that have been hidden from them. While the Archbishop of Dublin may drive me out of the Department of Health, he will not drive me out of politics. His interference, resulting in my resignation, will surely precipitate a general election and I will submit myself to the people again. I will run in direct opposition to the vassal Taoiseach in his own constituency. I am confident that the support which I receive will vindicate me in my struggle against the Bishops and make them look bad. I have no wish to damage the Church of which I am a member and by which I have been educated. I firmly believe that it is the autocratic Archbishop of Dublin rather than I, who is damaging the Church.

The Minister for Health, Dr Noël Browne, for all that he was an angular fellow, was a clear thinker and a straight talker – a plain blunt man. It was easy enough to capture his mindset as he approached his Ministerial demise. To divine what was the Archbishop's understanding of events – his mindset – is an altogether more challenging project. No single analysis entirely serves our purpose and therefore two conflicting hypotheses are proposed.

THE ARCHBISHOP'S MINDSET

The first hypothesis is that the Archbishop of Dublin believed implicitly that what he was doing was right. This analysis requires one to err on the side of charity, and to take an elasticated view of the evidence. Nevertheless, this interpretation would have been plausible a decade before when he was full of idealism, learning and charity. If he had continued in this mindset, his understanding of things in 1950 would have been something as follows.

The Minister for Health, while well meaning, is misguided and naive. He is determined to embark on a socialist path, or worse. The modernist tide, of which he is the spearhead, threatens to destroy the fibre of the Irish nation. I regret that the Minister must be destroyed but it is for the greater good. Since I am in the right and he is wrong, I am certain that history will vindicate me.

It is possible that, at this stage of the proceedings, he believed history would vindicate him and take a sanguine view of his actions: this optimism, however, did not endure. As he came towards the end of his life he realised that history would judge him harshly and his admirers would become a diminishing band – the penny had dropped.[155]

The alternative hypothesis regarding the Archbishop's mindset, although less edifying, is altogether more tenable.

I am the Archbishop of Dublin, God's main man in Ireland. True, there is the ageing Cardinal in Armagh but I sit in the metropolitan Archdioceses where the action is. I care little for this upstart Minister whom the herd have been foolish enough to elect. My power base, which I have carefully constructed over a decade, is secure. I control everything; the Church; the schools; the Universities; the health service. The power of my crozier terrifies the politicians. The Taoiseach is my creature. I can and will destroy anybody who dissents. Rome is watching. If I do this right the Red Hat, so unjustly denied me on several previous occasions by conniving enemies, may yet come my way. While I regard the Taoiseach as weak, he will serve as the instrument of my wrath and rid me of this nuisance Minister.

Acceptance of this analysis implies that the Archbishop had succumbed totally to the aphrodisiac of power and that it had corrupted him completely.

19

I Am the State

The memorandum was transmitted by the Taoiseach to be tabled at the drumhead court of the Bishops Standing Committee at the *Grande École*[156] at Maynooth. In the manner of all summary executions, events proceeded with dispatch. The Minister's memorandum having been submitted on March 28, the unsurprising fruit of Their Lordships deliberations was delivered to the Taoiseach without delay. The *coup de grace*, as was appropriate, was delivered not from Ferns, but from the real seat of Government at Drumcondra.

More than at any other time during his long reign must His Grace have been thinking, *L'état c'est moi.*

> The Archbishops and Bishops expressed grave disapproval of certain parts of the recently enacted Health Act 1947 especially those dealing with Mother and Child Services.

The Blacklist

The Hierarchy then proceed to enumerate those powers conferred by the Health Act which they look upon with 'grave disapproval'. These powers would enable the State:

> To provide for the health of all children.
>
> To treat their ailments.
>
> To educate them in regard to health.

To educate women in regard to motherhood.

To provide all women with gynaecological care.

That this quintet of proposals should be viewed by men of God 'with great disapproval' is entirely beyond normal comprehension. By their opposition to such a worthy list they have left many hostages to history. Furthermore, that the implementation of these measures should be obstructed by those disciples of Hippocrates sworn to look after the sick, is more than disappointing. Reason is turned on its head. Madness rules. A list of virtuous measures, basic to the Health Service of any civilised country becomes, by Episcopal whim, a vicious attack by a malign State on the rights of the individual. That the message of Jesus Christ could be so mutilated and manipulated by an Archbishop and his associates towards the objective of preserving their worldly power is a cause for despair. Even a cursory perusal of the Scriptures would have little difficulty in finding tracts to support the provision of each item on the Archbishop's extraordinary blacklist.

John Charles McQuaid's repeated use of the word 'all' ('all children', 'all women') in this passage is heavy with ideological import. It is as though, according to the blacklist, only some, not all, children should be the concern of the State. The thrust, he argues, should be one of charity rather than one of right. Let the State look after the scarcely relevant 'necessitous 10 per cent' – itself an absurdly small proportion not grounded in any statistical evidence. The rest, with the help of institutions and organisations mainly controlled by me and mine, can look after themselves. The message is clear, and music to the ears of the Irish Medical Association. The State should stay out of medicine – further evidence, if such be needed, of the Archbishop's alignment with the right wing.

Bad though it might be for the State to educate children in regard to health, 'to educate women in regard to motherhood' was, for the Archbishop of Dublin, the purest anathema. His attitude was, long before the world heard of such an aberration, Talibanesque – a charter for ignorance. The medical profession at this time was a supine enforcer of Catholic orthodoxy and sexual taboos, rather than a disseminator of biological insights. Many today will find it bizarre that anyone could object to the education of women, or anybody else, in matters biological – but Ireland was different then. Misogyny reigned and the Archbishop and his Church generally were its arch exponents.

An exemplar of institutionalised Church misogyny of the time, clearly remembered by this writer for his participation in the ritual as an altar boy, was the 'churching' of women. The postpartum woman presented herself alone and very publicly at the altar rails immediately after mass. The altar boy, while extinguishing the candles, noted her presence and informed the priest. Together they went with book and sprinkler and, by incantation and symbolic holy water, the woman was 'churched'. Although uncomprehending of the significance of the ritual at the time, and regretting his participation in it in retrospect, the altar boy came to realise that the Church, while much admiring of procreation, detested the act which brought it about, and devised a public ritual which would cleanse the woman of that taint.

Such was the atmosphere in which the Archbishop of Dublin, with the acquiescence of politics and medicine, could prohibit the education by the State of 'women in regard to motherhood'. It is indicative of the state of the nation at the time, that State policy with regard to 'gynaecological care' should fall within the ambit of a celibate clergy rather than of scientifically educated doctors – and it reflects poorly on the latter.

THE BILL OF RIGHTS

The list of 'rights', albeit on this occasion a mere quartet, which the Archbishop now states would be infringed by the new scheme, is no less extraordinary than the quintet of the blacklist.

The rights of the family.

The rights of the Church in education.

The rights of the medical profession'

The rights of voluntary institutions.

The Archbishop studiously avoids mention of the fact that participation in the Minister's scheme was to be entirely voluntary. He was perfectly at liberty to advise his flock to resist the diabolical temptation. This, if he had been convinced of the immorality of the scheme, would indeed have been an honourable course. If so convinced, he could have offered his followers 'blood, sweat and tears' in the cause of their salvation. He demeans his religion by subverting the laws of the state to enforce it. The evils which the Archbishop was fending off, however, were the product of his own imaginings as set out in the blacklist above. The Archbishop, instead of protecting 'the rights of the family' was doing precisely the opposite. He and his Episcopal colleagues were conspiring to prevent families from having a decent medical service.

It might be imagined that if 'the rights of the Church in education' were to be threatened, the menace would come from the cognate Government Department – Education. But the lazy State had completely surrendered to denominational education and thus, while paying lip service to the contrary, had copperfastened partition. The State had not yet produced a Minister for Education independent enough, or perhaps rash enough, to stand up to the Bishops as the Minister for Health was now doing.

It would be another generation before such a Minister for Education in the person of Donogh O'Malley[157] arrived. He, a man of some impetuosity, completely ignored the Hierarchy, and indeed most of his cabinet colleagues, with his impromptu announcement of free secondary education for all. He presented Their Lordships with that rarest of phenomena for them, a *fait accompli*. True to form the Bishops, still recoiling from the prospect of 'all children' being equally educated, opposed the measure but their objections were swept aside in a tide of popular acclaim. The worm was starting to turn. The price paid by Noël Browne had not been wasted and the generations who benefited from O'Malley' free education should be equally thankful to Browne. For the superstitious, however, the Bishop's curse appears still to have been operational – O'Malley died suddenly in 1968, not living to see the introduction of his epoch-making measure in 1969.

Using his power to support 'the rights of the medical profession' in their campaign to frustrate much needed progress has made McQuaid the laughing stock of history. He was, of course, intimate with the medical plutocracy and they shared with him a mutuality of purpose and a synergy of action in seeking to preserve their respective powers in the face of an encroaching State.

The Eunuch State

The word approve is much used in the Archbishops' letter to the Taoiseach. Approval is taken to mean by Their Lordship's house in Maynooth rather than by the elected house in Kildare Street.

> The Archbishops and Bishops desire to express once again approval of a sane and legitimate Health Service, which will properly safeguard the health of children and mothers.

It is noteworthy that nowhere in his letter to the Taoiseach does the Archbishop mention what had now become the *casus belli*, the means test. It is conveniently lost in the fog of war. He knows that he will lose credibility in the court of public opinion if it emerges that his insistence on a means test scuttled the scheme. Uncharacteristically he resorts to language which is bordering on the intemperate and is downright insulting to the Minister for Health. There is the clear implication that the Minister's Mother and Child Scheme (and perhaps by association the Minister himself) is not 'sane'.

In this national emergency only the Catholic Hierarchy, somewhat in the manner of generals in a banana republic, can save the nation from perdition. In these circumstances it is the Catholic oligarchy which must decide what is 'a sane health service' for the nation. Healthcare policy in a Catholic country is best formulated by us educated in the humanities. To leave it in the hands of crass scientists, sociologists and economists is self-evidently not 'sane'. We, the Princes of the Church, are the ones who see the big picture. We will step into the moral breach – *noblesse oblige*.

While there is no small arrogance in the Archbishop's use of the word 'sane', and lest the word on its own be insufficiently offensive, he amplifies it with adjective 'legitimate'. The Minister's scheme is not 'legitimate', or perhaps in language more apposite to the times, it is illegitimate. To be illegitimate was, in the eyes of the pious and prurient Ireland of mid-twentieth century, the gravest of stigmata. The Archbishop, an accomplished linguist, did not bandy words carelessly. The Minister's Mother and Child Scheme, in the eyes of the Hierarchy, was not legitimate: born out of holy wedlock it was a bastard.

The wedlock outwith which the Minister's scheme had the misfortune to be born was the happy union between the doyens of medicine and the Bishops. Towards the cavortings of this union the State was reduced to the role of an impotent observer – a eunuch State. The arrival of a politically virile third party into the *ménage,* in the person of Dr Noël Browne with his new ideas, was profoundly menacing to this domestic bliss. Life, if he was not dealt with, might never be the same again.

> The Hierarchy cannot approve of any scheme which in
> its general tendency, must foster undue control by the
> State in a sphere so delicate and so intimately concerned

with morals as that which deals with gynaecology or obstetrics.

It is not surprising that the Hierarchy should recoil in horror from anything which 'must foster undue control by the State'. Successive Governments, rather than fostering 'undue control', had lapsed into undue neglect. The impertinent Minister for Health was now seeking to re-assert the rights of the elected ones at the expense of the unelected – a kind of *coup d'état* in reverse. To prevent this democratic *démarche*, the Archbishop hatched his own coup. This event would be achieved by discrete and dignified manoeuvring. Although lacking the drama and vulgarity of the banana republic upheavals associated with such coups, it was nevertheless a grab by the right wing for control of the State.

In the Ireland of 1950 it might appropriately have been called a *coup d'église.*

Yet again the Archbishop stands logic on its head. History would judge that it was the Hierarchy and not the State which sought to practice 'undue control'.

> Neither can the Bishops approve of any scheme which must have for practical result the undue lessening of the proper initiative of individuals and associations and the undermining of self reliance.

Few would disagree with the Archbishop on the merits of encouraging 'initiative' and 'self-reliance'. Yet the essence of the Christian message is that we must help those who cannot help themselves. The Archbishop however operated a policy of 'do as I say, not as I do'.

Initiative is surely among the most admirable of qualities and this Minister for Health had shown plenty of it. In fact it was this faculty which now brought him into conflict with the Archbishop who is disingenuously, and with no small absurdity, posturing as a supporter and admirer of initiative. Up until then any such initiatives which had difficulty negotiating the filter of Drumcondra were discretely abandoned.

The Archbishop's resort to the noble attribute of 'self reliance' is perverse. Nothing undermines the 'self reliance' of an individual more than brain damage at birth, the result of inadequate obstetrical or neonatal services – precisely the services which the Minister was seeking to improve. Less dramatic but equally undeniable is the erosive influence of childhood poverty on subsequent health, mental and physical, with the consequent undermining of 'self reliance'. It is difficult to see how early detection and management of congenital abnormalities, a reliable enforceable immunisation programme, better childhood nutrition, and much else which the Minister sought to introduce, could do anything but improve rather than impair an individual's ability to achieve 'self reliance' later in life.

It was the Archbishop and his colleagues in the Hierarchy because of their quixotic fixation with, and narrow definition of, morals who were undermining 'self reliance'. Again, and for emphasis, nothing is more conducive to 'self reliance' than good physical and mental health, the foundations for which the Bishops were preventing the Minister from laying down.

If the Archbishop's argument made little sense with regard to the 'child' aspect of the scheme, it was equally bankrupt with regard to the 'mother' end of things.

Any mother, or indeed woman, of independent mind who was alive in 1950 and has had the good fortune to have endured, must surely burst out laughing at the notion of the Archbishop and the Hierarchy as the defenders of her 'initiative' and 'self reliance'. It was precisely the spectre of the emergence of these admirable attributes, so long dormant under the weight of the theocratic patriarchy, that seemed to be so exercising Their Lordships. Could it be that the Archbishop considered that 'initiative' and 'self reliance' were 'proper' only in the male of the species? In this regard medicine has profoundly altered its demographic in marked contrast to that of the Church. The latter, to the distress of many of its followers, remains as before, patriarchal, misogynistic and is increasingly sclerotic.

No Details Please

It was a feature of the Hierarchy's attitude throughout that they would not engage with the Minister in anything amounting to a true bilateral discussion of the points at issue. For the Archbishop of Dublin to engage with the Minister for Health was now *infra dignorum*. He would deal instead with the head of Government, the Taoiseach. In marked contrast to the Minister for Health, the Taoiseach was not a man who would point out to His Grace of Dublin the deficiencies of his argument: indeed of argument there was little.

> The bishops do not consider it is their duty to enter into an examination of the detailed considerations put forward by the Minister for Health in his memorandum

'The detailed considerations put forward by the Minister for Health' were a direct step by step rebuttal of the initial objections of the Hierarchy to the Mother and Child scheme. Such was the logic of that rebuttal that the Bishops were left without plausible counter argument. They, therefore, conveniently absolved themselves from 'the duty to enter into an examination' of the Minister's 'detailed' points. Like spoilt children in danger of losing the game they were grabbing all the marbles and running home.

It is sufficient for the Archbishop merely to state that the Minister for Health is guilty of a 'fallacy'. The docile Taoiseach and cabinet will accept that verdict without requiring 'an examination' of the evidence.

The Archbishop was not to be asked why it was more fallacious for the State to look after children's health than their education; why it was more fallacious to prevent maternal death than tubercular death or why it was fallacious to include more than 'the necessitous 10 per cent' in the scheme when 100 per cent were included in the scheme for children's allowances.

The Archbishop writes of the scheme as being 'set forth in vague and general terms'.

It is a measure of the extent to which the Archbishop is confounded by his lack of logical ammunition that he appears to contradict himself – a surprising lapse in a man of his precision and ability.

First he gives the Minister credit for 'the detailed considerations put forward' with regard to the Mother and Child Scheme. Then the Minister is accused of doing precisely the opposite, of not giving 'clear evidence of the details of implementation' and of only supplying Their Lordships with 'vague general terms'. The Bishops could not have it both ways. The Minister's position could not be, at one and the same time, 'detailed' and 'vague'.

The Archbishop then goes on to express his horror that the Mother and Child scheme 'has the appearance of conferring a benefit on the mothers and children of the whole nation'.

So egregious would this profligacy be that the Archbishop affects mild incredulity. Perhaps his scheme has only the 'appearance' (rather than the unthinkable reality) of proposing to inflict this iniquity on 'the whole nation'.

To the casual observer it might appear that 'conferring a benefit' on 'the whole nation' would be a better and a fairer thing to do than conferring it on a part; apparently not so. This is particularly surprising since the 'benefit' in question would improve the sorry lot of a great many mothers and children – surely a laudable objective and one to which the man from Nazareth was unlikely to take exception. The Archbishop, however, had allowed himself to be manoeuvred into a *cul de sac* from which he could only extricate himself by bullying rather than by logic. He is, in effect, now saying that what would be right for 10 per cent of the population would be morally wrong for the remaining 90 per cent. In any open forum of discussion he would, of course, get dismantled for such doublethink, but it worked fine when he was in conclave with the docile Taoiseach.

The inconvenient statistics of infant and maternal mortality, with which the Minister for Health had goaded the Hierarchy, did not feature in the Archbishop's riposte. It was deemed sufficient merely to say:

> The Hierarchy must regard the Scheme proposed by the Minister for Health as opposed to Catholic social teaching.

SEVEN PILLARS OF STRAW

The Archbishop now proceeds to rehearse, in a strange *diminuendo* format, as though running out of ideas, seven points of diminishing merit and increasing fatuity, in order to counter the Minister's assault on Catholic social (not moral) teaching.

> Firstly ... the State arrogates to itself ... control ... of education ... in the very intimate matters of chastity, individual and conjugal.

The verb to 'arrogate', to claim without right, is not part of the lexicon of common folk. Like all of the Archbishop's words it is chosen carefully. McQuaid sees the State, not as discharging its statutory functions with regard to the health of the people, but rather as arrogating – claiming something for itself without justification. The State was sticking its nose in where it did not belong.

CONJUGAL CHASTITY

Chastity was a big thing in mid-twentieth century Catholic Ireland – nothing wrong with that. Every child was taught, without having any idea what it was, that it was a good thing – and fair enough also. It is axiomatic, however, that one can have too much of a good thing and in classifying chastity into 'individual and conjugal' John Charles McQuaid would seem somewhat to be overstepping the mark. While there is no denying the societal benefits of what His Grace calls 'individual' chastity, his concept of the 'conjugal' variety – so clearly embedded in the Catholic teaching of the time – is more challenging.

If we abide by the standard definition of chastity as the abstention form sexual intercourse, the Archbishop's advocacy of the 'conjugal' variety was a difficult sell indeed. Viewed from the perspective of the twenty-first century, when even 'individual' chastity has become something of an eccentricity, the Archbishop's attempted imposition of the 'conjugal' variant seems somewhat beyond the realm of the outlandish. Such, however, was his position of power and authority that few questioned his occasional oxymoron. Most noteworthy among these must surely have been that combination of words – 'conjugal chastity'.

Thus we are treated to the spectacle of the Archbishop of Dublin hectoring not his flock but the Government on the surreal issue of 'conjugal' chastity. True, sexual activity could be tolerated by Their Lordships for the purposes of reproduction, but thereafter the unsavoury practice should be suspended, and in many instances was. To be fair, the Irish Catholic Bishops were not alone in this prudishness. Puritan elements in America were also making Hollywood look ridiculous. Prim and perfect couples, with twin beds separated by a specified measured distance, gave each other a Platonic peck before retiring. The male was at all times during this encounter required, in a touch of which the joyless McQuaid must have approved, to keep one foot on the floor. In America such foolishness was mere convention. In Ireland the Hierarchy, and not least he of the 'aphrodisiac cinema' from Galway, sought to make it Government policy.

PRIVATE LUXURY, PUBLIC SQUALOUR

It is clear that the Hierarchy believed that the State, if it was to have any role at all, should function only at the very margins of healthcare provision – confining its attentions to 'the necessitous 10 per cent'.

> Secondly ... Services ... properly ought to be and actually can be efficiently secured for the vast majority of the citizens by individual initiative and by lawful associations.

This is a recipe for what the Harvard economist Galbraith discordantly called 'private luxury, public squalor'.[158]

McQuaid does not, of course, mention the Church as such, but rather euphemises about 'lawful associations' – entities, the vast majority of which were owned and controlled by the Hierarchy, although significantly publicly funded. The Archbishop envisages a situation in which the State would disburse large amounts of public money to such 'lawful associations' – usually Catholic hospitals – to be applied at the discretion of those institutions, excused the intrusive tedium of normal public oversight. This, the public having only the vaguest idea of where such monies come from, served greatly to fortify the prestige and charitable profile of the Church.

While there is no denying the historic altruistic contributions of the many religious elements involved in Irish healthcare, these amounted to improvisations rather than a system. The Archbishop tries to put it across, ignoring damning statistics, that his 'lawful associations' had been satisfactorily catering for the health needs of the nation. In fact, to refer to the health of the nation as being managed by a system was to ignore the fact that little had been done, apart from the achievements of the present Minister Noël Browne, since the British left. Indeed it is not comforting to reflect that, if the British had not left, the situation would not have arisen. There would have been a comprehensive National Health Service, as in the separated six counties of Northern Ireland where it had been introduced to popular acclaim and, remarkably, without Episcopal demur.

Laissez faire, when applied to health services, does not have a happy history. For 'individual initiative' to work best there must be an overarching structure and framework and Government must be involved in this. In the absence of such intervention, the Archbishop's model, the comfortable classes by their undoubtedly admirable 'individual initiative' would be well looked after in dignified surroundings – 'private luxury'. The less well off, however, deprived of the advocacy at which the middle classes are so adept, would continue to endure what Noël Browne called 'the mark of the Poor Law', i.e. Galbraith's 'public squalor'.

PYRRHIC VICTORY

> Thirdly ... the State must enter unduly and very intimately into the life of patients, both parents and children and of doctors.

The Archbishop, in each of his enumerated seven points of attempted rebuttal, uses the expression 'this particular scheme'. He is, disingenuously, emphasising that it is only 'this particular scheme' which is a problem. The reason that this scheme was a problem for the Hierarchy was that this Minister refused to neuter it in response to Episcopal diktat, as had always happened before and in secret. By implication, therefore, it was not so much the scheme as its mentoring Minister which was the problem.

Precisely how much the State would have to do before it would be considered to 'enter unduly' into its citizen patients' affairs is not made clear by His Grace. It is difficult to conceive how anybody could think that a systemic scheme to improve the abominable state of children's health constituted undue interference. Yet this is the inescapable thrust of the Archbishop's argument. The issue, however, was one of control. Such benefits as might be provided for the less fortunate should be channelled not through the skeletal State but rather through the bloated Church. It would seem that the State would 'enter unduly into the lives' of people if it attempted to provide services universally regarded in civilised countries as normal. The Archbishop's battle cry was – the State at bay, the Church rampant.

Again we see the Archbishop advocating for the rights and privileges of doctors. This, although indefensible, was in understandable sympathy with his family background and his empathy with the doyens of medicine. History, however, might look more kindly on him if he had directed his advocacy towards those in more need of it. In this latter regard his victory over the Minister was a pyrrhic one. In addition, the historical reputation of the medical profession would have been better served if it had been spared this Episcopal advocacy.

TEA PARTY ECONOMICS

> Fourthly – To implement the scheme, the State must levy a heavy tax on the whole community, by direct or indirect methods, independently of the necessity or desire of the citizens to use the facilities provided.

Factually the Archbishop is correct – everything has to be paid for. Also, the Archbishop knew that the rich would always be able to look after themselves in salubrious establishments, and he is objecting to their being taxed to provide services for the less well off. His position was at variance with that of the founder of Christianity whom he purported to follow. He took an à *la carte* approach to the application of the Gospels and in this passage he is firmly ensconced in the corner of the moneychangers. He does not believe that 'the whole community' should be taxed to look after the less fortunate – an ignoble position for a senior churchman and a betrayal of the many sound rank and file clergy whose behaviour and lifestyles testified that they believed otherwise.

The Archbishop of Dublin is also advocating an extremely impractical à *la carte* approach to taxation. It is the exact antithesis of the Christian message that citizens should be taxed for the provision of a service only if they had the 'necessity or desire' to use it. This *naïveté*, as any Minister for Finance will know, is a formula for no revenue at all and no service at all – more Episcopal Tea Party economics.

With regard to 'the necessity or desire of the citizens to use the facilities provided' there can be no doubting either.

The 'necessity' was starkly illustrated by the national statistics with which the Minister had goaded the Hierarchy. The latter studiously ignored these numbers. The only statistic quoted by the Hierarchy throughout was 'the necessitous 10 per cent' and that was grasped out of thin air rather than being the fruit of any reproducible calculation. Why, if only 10 per cent of the citizens were 'necessitous', were the national rates of infant and maternal mortality so scandalous? Put at its simplest, the Archbishop, the Hierarchy and their medical abettors were prepared, against all the evidence, to deny the 'necessity' simply to keep the State out of medicine.

For the Archbishop to believe that 'the citizens' might not 'desire' to 'use the facilities provided' free would have required of him *na*ïveté of which few would consider him to have been afflicted. He knew that the people would flock to the service. He knew that 'State paid' general practitioners would implement the scheme, as they have always done when the State pay was attractive. He knew that new obstetric units would appear in State hospitals where he had less control. All in all, he anticipated, correctly, more State and less Church influence. To a man who had known the Church only in its rampant posture, and who regarded himself as Rome's main man in Ireland, this would have represented a severe reversal of fortune. Even if he saw the State's advance into medicine as inevitable – and it is extremely unlikely that he did – he was determined that the Church's retreat should not begin on his watch.

Happily for the Archbishop of Dublin, all the ingredients for a successful strike against the State's intrusion into medicine, and much else, were now at hand. He had the Taoiseach in his pocket. The cabinet were craven and terrified of the crozier. The medical leadership was tendentiously in support of his position. The population, weaned on a blend of nationalist Catholic jingoism and kept ignorant of the proceedings, would not question his actions. Into this mix, as if delivered to the Archbishop by providence, there now came this discordant Minister for Health who, like a straggling beast on the Serengeti, had detached himself from the protection of the herd and was ripe for exemplary destruction.

POLITICIAN MANQUÉ

> Fifthly – In implementing this particular scheme by taxation, direct or indirect, the State will, in practice, morally compel the citizens to avail of the services provided.

There is little difference between the content of this passage and the previous. The Archbishop appears to be repeating much of what he has said before and is bulking up his presentation by adding a scarcely relevant morsel.

John Charles McQuaid appears to have had a particular bee in his bonnet about taxation. A more worthy position for a Churchman would be to favour taxation of the rich within reason, as a device to redistribute to the less fortunate. This, indeed, would be orthodox Christian teaching and, paradoxically, found greater favour in more secular countries that it did in His Grace's theocratic Ireland. The Archbishop knew that, without revenue, the State would be impotent, and would not be in a position to challenge Church hegemony over his major medical institutions, or offer competition to them. His arguments are more like those to be expected from the leader of the opposition in parliament than from a Churchman. He is functioning more in political than in pastoral mode. Indeed, a few generations later, when Church careers became relatively less attractive, he might, formidably, have gone into politics.

Right now, however, the politician *manqué* had more power than the real one.

For the Archbishop to resort to the bogeyman of taxation was unworthy of his office but sat comfortably with his ideology. Nobody, except those paying none, likes taxation. The Archbishop here, however, brings to it a biblical aversion.[159] He was also preaching to the converted. The Government coalition was, with the exception of a rump of posturing leftists, made up mainly of conservatives led by a Taoiseach of like mind. Unworthy though it was, the introduction of the taxation ingredient into the argument was a clever ploy. It afforded disingenuous politicians an excuse to represent their opposition to the Minister for Health, not as abject fear of the crozier but rather as fiscal probity. In an absurd inversion of roles the politicians are worried about the Church's position while, in this passage, the Archbishop is talking only about money.

Self Reliance

> Sixthly – this particular scheme, when enacted on a nationwide basis, must succeed in damaging gravely the self reliance of parents.

The Archbishop's recruitment to his cause of the noble attribute of self reliance is bogus. Nobody, from Tea Party to Trotsky, is against self-reliance. The Irish people in particular, with their origins for the most part in the rural hinterlands, and with their history of cruel dispossession. have a visceral instinct for home ownership.[160] For example, the percentage of Irish people who struggle to pay off mortgages in order to own their own home is unrivalled elsewhere in Europe or beyond.[161] The later provision of free health services, altogether more comprehensive than what the Minister proposed in 1950, did nothing to diminish people's ambition to live in a house that they owned. The availability of public and rental housing did not 'succeed in damaging gravely the self reliance' which still drives people to own their own homes.

The same is true of healthcare. As the standards of publicly provided healthcare have improved in step with the national economy, the percentage of people paying for private health insurance has increased in proportion. At its peak, close to 50 per cent of the population, in spite of being entitled to a free hospital bed, paid for private health insurance. Never did the citizens contribute more to private health insurance than when, on a tide of national prosperity, free public services were at their best. And never were they more in need of a State safety net than when that tide went out. All of this is the opposite of what the Archbishop believed, or allowed himself, conveniently, to believe. The increased State involvement in healthcare and other areas did not cause the Irish instinct for independence and self sufficiency to atrophy. True, the people will take what they can get from the State but they are loath to allow themselves to become dependent upon it.

The Archbishop's argument is for private rather than publicly funded medicine – there is nothing wrong with that *per se*. There was, however, a lot wrong with a senior and powerful Churchman acting as an advocate for the private side, while actively obstructing the development of public services for those in dire need and who could never afford to pay for them. Few in his lifetime would venture to call the Archbishop a dog in the manger. History, however, is less inhibited.

STATUTORY INSTRUMENTS

> Seventhly – the State must have recourse, in greater part, to Ministerial regulations, as distinct from legislative enactments of the Oireachtas.

Analysis of this sentence reveals the extent to which the Hierarchy felt empowered to interfere in the minutiae of the running of the State.

When an Act is signed into law by the President, it contains clauses which give the relevant Minister certain discretion that he may exercise using 'Statutory Instruments' (under the Statutory Instruments Act, 1947, such instruments are defined as 'an order, regulation, rule, scheme or bylaw made in exercising the power conferred by the statute'). It is doubtful that the State could function without such statutory instruments – for example, 791 were issued in 2012. Certainly an active minister would be completely hamstrung if denied 'recourse' to such instruments. The Archbishop sought to deny the Minister for Health that 'recourse'. Statutory instruments are used for the fine tuning and detail of an act of law. It was not so much the bones of the act that the Hierarchy feared but rather the meat that the Minister for Health might put on them.

The Archbishop thus sought to deny the Minister for Health his statutory prerogative in the implementation of the Health Act. The Minister was to have no discretion. The Archbishop had insisted, in the first paragraph of his memorandum, that every minute detail must be written down 'in a legally binding manner and in an enactment of the Oireachtas'. He would, no doubt, expect to have sight and oversight of every detail as he had in the divisive and partitionist 1937 constitution. The Archbishop feared that once the skeleton of the act was in place – what he called 'the principle' – the minister, by 'recourse' to 'regulations', could enable doctors to provide services and advice to patients of which Their Lordships did not approve. Catholic teaching 'must' be enshrined in detail 'in an enactment of the Oireachtas'.

HIS GRACE'S *COUP DE GRACE*

His Grace of Dublin, triumphant, is finishing his meander with an appropriate flourish – indeed, one might say, a *coup de grace*.

He is smug and he has reason so to be. His enemy is routed and his grip on the levers of State is complete.

> Finally – The Bishops are pleased to note that no evidence has been supplied in the letter of the Taoiseach that the proposed Mother and Child Scheme advocated by the Minister for Health enjoys the support of the Government.

The Archbishop is now indulging himself in the fiction that the Mother and Child Scheme was never really Government policy at all. The whole debacle had in fact been some kind of mistake – a misunderstanding. The main parties to the affair (not the Minister for Health who is now a non-person), the Hierarchy and the Government, are now in agreement and, praise the Lord, 'The Bishops are pleased'.

Since he, finally, was forced to face the issue, the Taoiseach has been backpedalling furiously. He is frantically, and dishonourably, seeking to disassociate himself and his cabinet colleagues from the misguided proposal of his maverick Minister. He is allowing the Archbishop to exculpate himself of meddling, on the pretext that the Mother and Child Scheme was never really Government policy. The scheme was no more than an obsession of the Minister for Health. Now, alas, as a result of Church and medical chicanery the scheme no longer 'enjoys the support' of the cabinet. The abandoned Minister is a dead man walking.

From the triumphalism of his opening sentence – 'the Bishops are pleased' – the Archbishop now launches into unctuous and patronising mode.

> Accordingly the Hierarchy have firm confidence that it will yet be possible, with reflection and calm consultation, for the Government to provide a scheme which, while it affords due facilities for those whom the State, as guardian of the common good, is rightly called

upon to assist, will none the less respect, in its principles and implementation, the traditional life and spirit of our Christian people.

He proceeds to affect concern for the standards of a health service, improvements to which he and his medical abettors have been conspiring to sabotage. Implausibly, he assures us that the Bishops are in favour of a good public health service – but would the State please confine itself to the 'necessitous 10 per cent'.

Not only are the Bishops 'pleased' but the Hierarchy have 'firm confidence' in the course that events are now taking. 'God's in his heaven, all's right with the world'.[162]

Next the Archbishop addresses himself, having driven the ship of public health services on to the rocks, to a mission of mercy and salvage. There must now be a period of 'reflection and calm consultation'. So well would the politicians reflect that, in the face of any Episcopal disapproval, they would for generations be reduced to a gelatinous quiver. Normally of short memory, they carried the trauma of the episode for half a century. Not until the new century, with Church power a mere shadow of its former self, would a later Taoiseach[163] in a show of populist bravado and now at no risk of crozier induced trauma, posture at standing up to the Hierarchy – a melodramatic and much belated closing of the stable door.

Consultation would now revert to the traditional form of a nod from Drumcondra.

It is, of course, entirely right that any health service should accommodate local traditions and sensitivities. The Archbishop, however, does not feel disposed or able to enlighten us as to which principles of the founder of Christianity would be violated by the Minister's scheme.

For John Charles McQuaid to don the cloak of concern for 'traditional life' is worthy of Hans Christian Andersen. The Archbishop lived, not over the ample shop in Drumcondra, but, fairy-tale like, in millionaires' Dalkey-Killiney.[164] By way of clarifying this grandiosity, his house, which subsequently became a diplomatic residence, was on the rental market in 2007 for €216,000 *per annum*. It was sold (in need of refurbishment) in 2015 for €4,065,000.[165] Thus lived the man who accused the Minister for Health of endangering 'traditional life'.

The Minister, in contrast, was a true exemplar of traditional life. He learned to speak Irish and went to live in a cottage in Connemara. With regard to power politics, however, he was reduced to the role of pundit rather than practitioner. His historical legacy has enjoyed an advantage denied the Archbishop. As with all who die young he was removed from power before it had time to corrupt him.

20

CONTROL THEN AND NOW

The appointment of senior doctors to major hospitals, and particularly the fairness of the procedures involved, is a matter of fundamental importance with regard to standards and morale. Up to mid twentieth century, and still to a significant degree, this has been controlled by Church interests. As Government began increasingly to invest in health services, a system of Statutory, as distinct from Voluntary Hospitals began to emerge under secular governance. The Bishops did not control senior medical appointments to such institutions and this caused them alarm.

While this anxiety applied partly to general practitioners it is also reflective of the Bishops' attitude to hospital appointments. The spectre of 'lay bureaucrats' having a role, indeed a determining one, in hospitals outwith the control of the Bishops and their beholden senior doctors, loomed large. Control of what was happening in medicine was becoming more slippery in the hands of Their Lordships. Notwithstanding their academic excellence, there was alarm that senior doctors could now be appointed who might not pass the Bishops' test. There was the alarming possibility that what had heretofore been determined by mitre, might now be determined by the less controllable parameter of merit.

SAUCE FOR THE GOOSE NOT SAUCE FOR THE GANDER

Such new senior medical appointments to hospitals that we are calling secular, increasing in number and prestige, became the responsibility of a State entity lumbered with the rather drab moniker 'the Local Appointments Commission'.[166] The Commission was responsible for a wide range of appointments across the full range of the public service, mundane and exotic. The doyens of medicine, whom we described earlier as being not without pretension, did not take kindly to being lumped in with such vulgarians.

The Local Appointments Commission however had a stout record of independence and integrity. The very purpose for which it had been set up by the new State was to avoid nepotism and political jobbery and in this, for all its drabness, it had succeeded admirably.

An appointments procedure sporting the ostensibly desirable attributes of independence, integrity and untainted by nepotism and jobbery was however not considered suitable for appointing senior doctors to Church-owned hospitals which had long enjoyed a free rein in appointing those who scored highly in the category of 'suitability'. The criterion of 'suitability', when applied adroitly by a suitably chosen interview board, could be deployed with good effect and the utmost respectability against the less pious, the unconnected and those 'educated in institutions in which we have no confidence'.

The Local Appointments Commission (now called the Public Appointments Service) has always been looked upon with condescension by the urbane metropolitan cognoscenti in Medicine. Along with their Episcopal allies they conspired together, with success, to keep their appointments procedures for consultant doctors 'in house' and free from the intrusions of 'lay bureaucrats'. The Bishops and their senior medical allies decided that the system which was impartially appointing city and county managers, engineers, librarians and many other elements of the backbone of the developing nation, would have no place in appointing senior doctors to the hospitals they controlled. They would abide by their own procedures and suitably constitute their own interview boards for senior posts. Indeed His local Lordship might preside as chairman of such senior medical appointments boards, these latter sometimes referred to at the time and long afterwards, without batting an eyelid, as 'the Bishop's committee'. Doubtless His Lordship on such occasions affected a benign neutrality. His crozier however was never far away and a compliant and beholden medical elite rarely made it necessary for him to resort to *force majeure.*

The Church did, it should be acknowledged, own the hospitals and felt entitled to this control, but this regime of in house control has endured, notwithstanding that such institutions are now completely dependent on public funding.

Thus the average taxpayer of today will not be aware that he funds two separate and very different consultant doctor appointments systems, one statutory and fully answerable to democratic scrutiny, the other improvised and less so. He will be equally unaware that his government continues to acquiesce in this. An aspiring young candidate, who comes early for interview, as is indeed the habit of all careful candidates, could find himself closeted in the antechamber with one whose cousin or uncle or brother-in-law is participating in, or indeed presiding over, events within.

This is in marked contrast to the austerity of the Public Appointments Service gig, presided over by a formidable lay and disinterested chairperson nominated by the service, and a diverse panel of specialist doctors with no axe to grind. The unconnected outsider of merit might better fancy his chances in such a place.

This was the Episco-Medical alliance in action and it has continued to frustrate the emergence of a common selection procedure for public service consultant doctors. It is doubtful that this ambiguity would have survived if Noël Browne had endured.

ARTICLE 44: A TWO-WAY STREET

It will seem extraordinary to some today that the Minister for Health in 1950 had to explain to the Hierarchy why he could not countenance religious discrimination in the public appointments system. The lazy State, however, while funding hospitals and other institutions of both the Roman and Reformed traditions, had lapsed into a policy of *laissez faire* which allowed both, Article 44 of the Constitution[167] notwithstanding, to discriminate in favour of their own.

Some will argue, and well they might, that the Archbishop's *bête noir* Protestant Churches were not above reproach in such matters. Their hegemony was in retreat, however, while that of Drumcondra was at its zenith and he lacked magnanimity. They can, therefore, be more easily forgiven for circling the wagons. Their hospitals, indeed, were no slouches when it came to defending their much trumpeted 'ethos'. Towards the preservation of that understandably treasured ethos, nursing recruits were mainly drawn from the urban mercantile class and from the county set and invariably kicked, to use the Caledonian idiom, with the right foot.

The Matron of such establishments, as she selected nubile nursing material to preserve her ethos, was no more concerned than was the Archbishop of Dublin with Article 44. Indeed, she equally could resort to the same Article 44 which states that 'every religious denomination shall have the right to manage its own affairs'. Constitutions, it would seem, are somewhat like scriptures and can be cited selectively to suit the purpose of devils,[168] Government Ministers, Archbishops – and Matrons.

TAXATION WITHOUT REPRESENTATION

We have already noted that the expression 'Voluntary Hospital', while being semantically correct in former times, and having a noble history, is a misnomer in the modern epoch.

The Archbishop of Dublin, John Charles McQuaid, had a spectacular gift for raising funds, often from the State, and dressing up their disposal in institutions which he or others of the Hierarchy controlled, as Catholic Church largesse. This 'largesse', for example in the funding of Church-controlled hospitals, often passed for charity, as did the hospitals so controlled pass as 'voluntary'. This perception was reinforced by the fact that the disbursers of these funds in such hospitals were most often highly visible, efficient, kindly and altruistic nuns in the true Nightingale tradition. The funding of such entities, however, came increasingly from the public purse.

The Archbishop of Dublin envisaged a hospital service in which the State would continue to cough up increasingly large amounts of public money and he and his colleagues, through their various agents, would vicariously control its application. While it is readily conceded that the nuns were thrifty in the usage of such monies, and today such historic thrift is hankered after with naïve sentimentality, the structure nevertheless represented taxation without representation – the citizen of the State was taxed to pay, the Bishops controlled.

One might have expected a man of the Archbishops erudition and accomplishment, although not significantly weighed down by democratic baggage himself, to have known that the combination of democracy and 'taxation without representation' was an oxymoron. Eventually, as Oscar Wilde said of the wallpaper,[169] one of them would have to go.

While the Department of Finance with its draconian powers has always been more than assertive in enforcing the 'taxation' end of things upon the citizen, the Department of Health, because of Church ownership of the hospitals, had an altogether more difficult task in asserting the 'representation' on the citizens' behalf. The civil service mandarins, although right minded, have always had the greatest difficulty in penetrating the inner financial workings of certain Church-controlled medical institutions. The Minister for Health of 1950, however, was about to beef up the 'representation' and this, as much as the non-issue of the means test, was probably what raised the Archbishop's hackles. While the politicians of 1950 were exuberant in expressing their fealty to the Church, it is not in the nature of the species to yield credit for their pork barrel spending to others – even to Archbishops.

The Archbishop of Dublin was stealing not only the politicians' money but also their clothes: it could not last.

It is the duty of civil service mandarins to see to it that public monies, allocated for a specific purpose, are applied accordingly. This is particularly important in the health service where the amounts involved are gargantuan. This implied a level of intrusive micromanagement – or 'representation' – odious to institutions controlled by Their Lordships. This writer, at meetings on more than a few occasions, witnessed management of such institutions bristle with indignation at the temerity of sound public officials sent in to such places to effect oversight of how public money was spent. It is not so much that impropriety was suspected but rather that the intrusion was powerfully resented. The Archbishop's position was that the State should do the dirty work of taxation and his 'lawful associations' would reap the kudos of spending.

The Archbishop, a shrewd contriver at extracting the money, did not see that, inevitably, this success would erode his control. He still believed in the free lunch.

Gradually more secular hospitals, of critical mass and penetrable financial arrangements, began to enjoy the favour of the mandarins. Certain of these have become significant on occasion blooming out of old Poor Law workhouses.[170] One can only imagine the despair with which His Grace, if he had lived to see it, would have viewed the rise and rise of St James's Hospital – the main teaching hospital of his unloved Trinity College Medical School and more than a match for his favoured Catholic institutions.

But worse still has happened – the Archbishop's ultimate nightmare come true. His beloved signature project whose name is emblematic of his time, Our Lady's Hospital for Sick Children (1956), is tired, scientifically isolated, and has run its course. Frantic, wasteful,[171] pantomime efforts to shoe horn the replacement institution into the constricted site of one of His Grace's flagship hospitals, the Mater Misericordiae, were penetrated and ruptured not by doctors, politicians or Bishops, but by the horse-sense of town planners. His Grace, from wherever he now views events, will have to 'suffer the little children'[172] going to that place he detested most and in whose denizens he had 'no confidence' – St James's of Trinity College.

Surely the unkindest cut of all.

21

RESIGNATION

The Hierarchy were not accustomed to being presented with such impertinent truths as those with which the Minister was now hammering them. Theirs was a world where the difficult questions were disposed of by the teaching that such matters were not meant to be understood. This is fair enough to a degree but, taken too far, can make one look silly. It is reasonable to tell people that profound theological mysteries must be taken as a matter of faith. To ask them to believe, however, that the absence of a means test was an affront to God was another matter entirely. This, with the logic of Caligula, was what the Archbishop of Dublin was trying to put across. The moral ramifications of the Minister's scheme were of such profound import and complexity, the Archbishop would have people believe, as to be beyond their powers of comprehension and the Bishops, who always knew best would guide them. Indeed, the argument went, were not all the politicians in agreement with the Hierarchy. And finally it was well known, and he stated it himself, that in spite of all his disagreement with Their Lordships, the Minister was still a devout Catholic.

The only conclusion possible: the Bishops must be right.

GALILEO

In order to assert themselves Their Lordships would do a Galileo[173] on the Minister. As their antecedents had destroyed

Galileo for the uncomfortable logic of his science, so they would now destroy the Minister for the inconvenient logic of his argument.

Galileo, like the Minister for Health, was guilty of what has become known as 'thinking outside the box'[174] – an indulgence little favoured by the Catholic Church at the time of Galileo in 1630, particularly out of fashion in the Ireland of 1950, and indeed achieving little traction with the Church managers as we advance into the twenty-first century. Supporting Copernicus'[175] theory that the earth revolved around the sun, Galileo fell foul of the Church, whose sages insisted that scripture said otherwise and accused Galileo of heresy. He was, accordingly, summoned to Rome, tried by the Holy Inquisition, and found guilty of being 'vehemently suspect of heresy' and, lucky to escape with his head, spent the rest of his days under house arrest.

The parallels between the fate of Galileo and that of the Minister for Health of 1950 are irresistible. True, the Minister, unlike Galileo, was spared the rigours of arduous travel: when summoned he had only to cover the two kilometres north to Drumcondra. When he arrived there, however, he encountered, as Galileo had done centuries before, the powerful sages of the Church in full groupthink mode. The motivation for the destruction of both 'outside the box' thinkers was identical. Groupthinkers and 'outside the box' thinkers make extremely unhappy bedfellows. The life of the former is comfortable and tranquil while the latter, with his fermenting mind and his often inconvenient analysis, arouses suspicion, antipathy and sometimes fear. As Dr Noël Browne found out, life is hard for the 'outside the box' man.

The Catholic Bishops of 1950 were groupthinkers *par excellence* and so it has, with some exceptions, continued since. They exhibited the classical feelings of invulnerability and moral rectitude typical of the syndrome. Was not their boss in Rome infallible? True the Pope was only considered infallible when speaking *Ex Cathedra* on matters of faith and morals. It was, however, on this very matter of faith and morals, that the Hierarchy based their bogus objections to the Mother and Child Scheme.

The behaviour of the Hierarchy towards the Minister for Health lacked even the legitimacy of those who condemned Galileo. The latter, at least, were part of the temporal Government apparatus of the Papal State and were abiding, albeit odious and ignorant, by official procedure. They issued an official judgement. Furthermore, the Church sages of 1630 actually believed that the sun went around the earth. It seems that the sages of 1630, while misguided, were acting in good faith and issued their verdict in accordance with most accepted wisdom of the time. The Hierarchy of 1950, in contrast, while having no statutory role, were now issuing the Government with its riding orders in regard to taxation and proposed legislation policy. Also, much of what went on would have remained buried for a generation if the Minister had not blown the gaff.

It has to be concluded that the Hierarchy, in destroying the Minister for Health because of their insistence on a means test, did not act in good faith. They did not believe in their hearts that the scheme was wrong.

Matters are now proceeding apace. The idealistic Noël Browne as Minister for Health is completely isolated in Cabinet. His resistance to the Bishops has made him a political liability. Only the manner of his departure remains to be determined. He was not one to go quietly.

ENTER McBRIDE

Mr Sean McBride, Minister for External Affairs, was Noël Browne's Clann Na Poblachta party leader and had nominated him to the Cabinet – something which he was now coming deeply to regret. The union between these two awkward fellows, while previously business-like, has become dysfunctional in the extreme. At this stage the only thing which they had in common was their idiosyncrasy of speech. McBride, who was reared in Paris, paraded his exotic credentials by rolling his Rs, but in a manner which would not have caused him to be mistaken for a man who hailed from the banks of the Suir. Browne, educated in England, although not quite exhibiting an 'ascendency' accent, stopped well short of a brogue – *prima donnas* both.

McBride, according to Browne's account in his memoir, made every effort to persuade him to abandon his principled objection to a means test. Browne, however, was not endowed with McBride's pragmatism. The latter, having completely caved in to the crozier, decided, in the interest of his own political preservation, that Browne must go. McBride denounced him at a party meeting on 17 March 1951, to wide support – the leftish elements in Clann Na Poblachta were no less scared of the Bishops than everybody else.

On 10 April 1951 McBride handed Noël Browne a letter demanding that he resign as Minister for Health stating:

> The creation of a situation where it is made to appear that a conflict exists between the spiritual and temporal authorities is always undesirable. In the case of Ireland, it is highly damaging to the cause of national unity and should have been avoided.

This is five star hypocrisy. McBride, who had been wedded to the gun rather than to parliamentary methods, had, in an earlier incarnation, been no less than the Chief of Staff of the thoroughly violent and undemocratic rump 'Irish Republican Army' (IRA). He, who had thus done so much to alienate northern Unionists, now has the gall to accuse the Minister for Health of 'damaging the cause of national unity'. Furthermore, he seeks to camouflage his capitulation to the Bishops on the Mother and Child scheme with the anodyne statement:

> I wish to state categorically that the establishment with the minimum delay of such services in the freest sense

of the word and with the least impediment possible has
been my earnest wish....

Lack or inadequacy of means should not deprive any
mother or child from receiving the best possible medical
care and attention that money and science can provide.

Now the man who wrote this was, out of fear of the Bishops
and out of political expediency, abandoning the Minister
for Health who proposed to provide that 'care and attention'.
McBride knew that resistance to the Mother and Child
Scheme would not be judged kindly by history. In his efforts
to exculpate himself, one might be forgiven for thinking that
the Archbishop, not McBride, had written much of the letter.
For all his posturing as a great liberal, McBride was as much
in the pocket of the Archbishop as was the Taoiseach, but he
lacked the latter's disarming and honest frankness about being
so. McBride, dishonourably, was seeking to run with the hare
and hunt with the hounds – the hounds of God.

Up until the time of receiving McBride's letter
unceremoniously dumping him, Noël Browne had been
measured in what he wrote; decorum ruled. The letter, however,
ignited a spark in the tinderbox that he had become, causing
him to abandon all inhibition and launch into an unseemly
tirade of personal abuse of a kind politicians rarely commit to
paper. A few examples of this will suffice.

Your letter is a model of two faced hypocrisy and
humbug so characteristic of you. Your reference to the
conflict between the spiritual and temporal authorities
will occasion a smile among the many people who
remember the earlier version of your kaleidoscopic self.

Expediency is your sole yardstick, and to expediency
you are prepared to sublimate all principles, sacred and
profane.

It is my fervent hope that the destiny of my country will never be placed fully in your hands because it would, in my view, mean the destruction of all those ideals which are part and parcel of our Christian democracy.

I have bidden farewell to your unwholesome brand of politics.

Doubtless Noël Browne felt better having unburdened himself of such vitriol, but the outburst does little for his credibility. Also, his onslaught is directed at Sean McBride while his main adversary was always the Archbishop of Dublin. He used the former as a whipping boy for the latter. It was easier to assail the 'kaleidoscopic' man of two faces and much 'humbug', than to take on John Charles McQuaid who, although perhaps less 'kaleidoscopic', would be considered by few today to be free of the said 'humbug'.

On Thursday, 11 April 1951, Noël Browne resigned as Minister for Health. On the following day *The Irish Times* fearlessly published the full correspondence surrounding the controversy, which, flouting all convention, he had released to them. His resignation shared the front page of the paper with the sacking of a man no less stubborn. General Douglas MacArthur was fired by President Truman for insubordination – he wanted to bomb China in the Korean War.

Noël Browne never held cabinet office again.

It is noteworthy that, even in this extremity, and at the very point of his destruction by the Archbishop of Dublin, the Minister should still extol the virtues of 'Christian democracy'. This latter, however, was in little danger from McBride who was soon afterwards dumped by the electorate and he never held political office again. His 'kaleidoscopic' past forgotten, he reinvented himself as an international champion of liberal causes. The Archbishop, however, was more durable: a poor exemplar of the Christian ethic, and entirely spared of democratic pretension, he remained a burden on the nation and on his Church for a further twenty years.

In his resignation letter Noël Browne stated:

> As a Catholic I accept the rulings of Their Lordships without question.

The Irish Times wrote: 'A new scheme – with a means test – will now be necessary.'

Mortally wounded the coalition Government limped on until a general election on 30 May 1951. A new minority Fianna Fáil Government under de Valera assumed office on 13 June 1951.

The ghost of the Mother and Child Scheme had, however, not gone away. The new Minister for Health, Dr James Ryan, re-inherited the poisoned chalice so fortuitously snatched from him in 1947.

A superstitious mind might be tempted to wonder if the Mother and Child Scheme were jinxed – if it carried, in the manner of the breaching of the tomb of Tutankhamen,[176] some kind of curse. Its first promoter, the estimable Dr Conor Ward (1947), fell foul of the Internal Revenue in his personal affairs and was unseated by the scandal. Now, in its second coming (1950), the scheme along with its second Minister Dr Noël Browne offended 'the Archbishops and Bishops', and the scheme and its Minister were duly unseated. The third Minister to tackle the problem – by now an extremely toxic chalice – was Dr James Ryan of Fianna Fáil who took over Health after the Costello Government fell (1951). He had been somewhat cavalier in not consulting Drumcondra before promulgating the third iteration of the Mother and Infant Scheme – still without a means test. He was persuaded by the pragmatic de Valera and his able deputy Sean Lemass to save himself from the fate of his two predecessors only by reluctantly accepting and incorporating a means test. The curse remained however.

The Fianna Fáil Government fell before Ryan could implement the scheme. It finally came into law, with a means test, in 1956 under Costello's Minister Tom O'Higgins.[177]

After nine years, four Ministers and much dirty tricks, the means test was back. The lesson had been learned.

No Contrition

In considering if the institutional Catholic Church is contrite regarding the damage it did to the Minister for Health, to the Health Service, to its followers, to the country and to itself, we might again resort to Galileo.

The great astronomer, in order to save himself from the standard chastisement of burning at the stake, recanted his 'heresy'. Of course, he still knew that he was right and that the earth went around the sun, but in his further extensive writings in captivity he stayed away from the taboo subject of the heavenly bodies.

For the Church to concede grudgingly that it might not have been entirely right about Galileo took some time – 350 years.

Long after the scientific world accepted that Galileo was right, the sages of the Church held tough, explaining their position with slippery Jesuitical doublethink. The line was that while Galileo might have been right, the Church, in all the circumstances prevailing, had not really been wrong in the way in which it had dealt with him. Even this half-baked admission took 200 years. After another century Galileo was, still using the language applied to criminals, pardoned. But still there was, in the verbiage of the Four Courts, no admission of liability. The Red Hat sages of the Church were not, and could not be seen to be, wrong. The conviction of Galileo was not wrong or unjust: it was simply, as an appeal court might say in order to save the face of the system, unsafe.

Eventually, in 1992, Pope John Paul II, possibly out of empathy with his fellow Polish countryman Copernicus, who started all the trouble, cleared the great astronomer Galileo of all wrongdoing. Even the most careful scrutiny of his speech, however, will have difficulty in finding the words – sorry, we were wrong.

The Minister for Health, Dr Noël Browne, refusing to recant, was burned at the political stake and for the rest of his public life was condemned to the role of a malcontent sniping from the wings of politics. The triumphalist John Charles McQuaid, having scored such a happy victory for the Church and having drawn approbation from the ultra-conservative Pope Pious XII, must surely have thought that he was on his way to the much coveted Red Hat. How he would have loved to have used his formidable persuasive powers on his fellow Cardinals, and then shuffled in to the Sistine Chapel to elect a safe Pope. It was not, however, to be. A man of such Machiavellian bent as McQuaid is never without enemies and some, within his own tent, spiked his guns and he was repeatedly passed over for the ultimate piece of clerical headgear[178] – he had to settle for a mere mitre.

Following his victory over Noël Browne there was an immediate and worrying straw in the wind for the Archbishop. In the subsequent general election precipitated by the Church-Medical conspiracy the Minister (alas now only Dr Browne) topped the pole in the constituency he shared with the Taoiseach, beating the latter into a poor second. The political vassal of Drumcondra, although humiliated, survived and, his affectation of reluctance notwithstanding, would return later to the Taoiseach's office. The Archbishop cannot have been pleased by the poll. He would have known that the shifty dispensers of red hats in Rome would have an eye for such things.

As for a Galileo-style acknowledgement that 'we were wrong', there is time enough – only sixty-five years have passed.

BURNING LETTERS

It is a matter of public record that there was significant support for the Minister from trade unions and from the left generally. Furthermore, more than a few doctors were in favour of the scheme. Such was the squinting windows[179] atmosphere of the time, however, that much of this remained covert. While a number of doctors sided publicly with the Minister against the Hierarchy, few who depended for a living on a clinical practice thought it wise to do so. In the land of Captain Boycott a raised voice or even a raised eyebrow in the pulpit, could empty the waiting room fast.

In his memoir, written many years later, the Minister writes of the many letters of support which he received from doctors around the country. It is not comforting to reflect on his fear that the writers could be compromised by discovery of such correspondence. On his resignation he destroyed all the letters. This was a reprehensible act of historical vandalism. It was furthermore much out of character for this Minister. Perusal of relevant files in the National Archives of Ireland shows him to be punctilious at documentation. Perhaps it is true that the Minister feared a McCarthyite witch hunt against his supporters. It was, after all, the 1950s and McCarthy and Hoover in America had an able *alter ego* in Ireland in John Charles McQuaid.

Dr Noël Browne violated standard administrative procedure when, immediately on his resignation in April 1951, he released confidential departmental files to the press, specifically *The Irish Times*. He did this in an effort to vindicate his position and many would agree that he was justified in doing so. He was, as we have stated, setting the historical record. But why then did he, according to his own account, destroy the extensive documentary support he said he had received – evidence which would have further served to vindicate his position? If such voluminous supporting correspondence from doctors existed, he did not have to publish it immediately with the rest: it should however, have been left in the files for the historical record. Indeed, it is fair to point out in this context that the Minister's adversary, the Archbishop of Dublin, Dr McQuaid, left, in the

Dublin Diocesan Archive, voluminous material at least some of which, he must have known, would cause him not to be judged kindly by history. The destruction of documents never lends credibility to an argument, and if such letters existed in quantity the Minister undermined his case by destroying them.

22

SUPERFICIAL AND DEEP EXCELLENCE

Dr Noël Browne, as Minister for Health in 1950, sought to produce excellence in maternity and child care and undoubtedly, incrementally, to expand such excellence into other areas of medical practice. The emergence of excellence in the public healthcare system, particularly in hospitals, always causes anxiety on the private side, as it caused anxiety in the Archbishop of Dublin in the case under discussion. This fear is ill founded. Such public excellence, often achieved at great effort, is extremely difficult to sustain. Trade union hegemony, indifferent health service management and structures, gyrating national economic fortunes and the lobbying of the private sector all conspire towards a grinding mediocrity.

The Minister for Health of 1950, however, had already produced, and sustained, excellence in dealing with the nation's main health problem, tuberculosis. The population voted with its feet in acceptance of the new free service and so they would again with regard to obstetrics, gynaecology and child services, if the public service were allowed to achieve a satisfactory standard.

The medical establishment, therefore, particularly metropolitan elements towards the upper end of the food chain, had a most un-Hippocratic antipathy towards the Minister's efforts to produce excellence in public obstetric and paediatric services. This was for two reasons.

The first relates to the perennial tension between excellence and mediocrity in Irish healthcare. There was the fear that public excellence might expose private mediocrity.

Excellence in healthcare is extremely expensive: it requires more equipment, more and better trained staff and more investment generally. The matter is further complicated by the fact that, in hospitals, there are two kinds of excellence which might be characterised as superficial and deep. Superficial, or domestic, excellence is that which is immediately apparent to the casual observer – housekeeping, catering, ample space, lack of crowding etc. Deep, or scientific, excellence is embedded in the system, is not seen by the casual observer and is validated only by penetrating audit.[180] While scientific excellence is expensive and less visible, domestic excellence is affordable and up front for all to see. In Ireland, public hospitals, even those achieving scientific excellence, have, not infrequently been cursed by domestic mediocrity. Private institutions, by contrast, have sometimes masked scientific mediocrity by domestic excellence.

It is cheaper to provide an environment of creature comforts than one of twenty-four hour scientific intensity.

The argument, as presented here, was belatedly vindicated by events – and, as luck would have it, by events in the very field of maternity and neonatal services under discussion. The complications of obstetrical and neonatal medicine are stark indeed and are always, whether avoidable or otherwise, emotionally charged. Private maternity units of domestic excellence, but questionable scientific depth, attracted the attention of predatory lawyers. A feeding frenzy of litigation, with awards out of all proportion to the resources of the Irish economy, followed. Private obstetrical entities were now being proven unsafe, not by the medical denizens who prospered therein, but by lawyers. Unable to afford the expensive environment required for safety, and therefore unable to insure themselves, such units began to close. On occasion such closures were accompanied by public outcry and lobbying[181] by those who appreciated the domestic excellence, but could not gauge the scientific risk.

At the time of writing there is no private maternity facility in Ireland. Furthermore, private hospitals providing general services are not subjected by law to the exacting auditing standards visited upon public institutions by the Health Information and Quality Authority (HIQUA).

The second reason the medical establishment and their patrons, the Bishops, felt threatened by the prospect of excellent public services was more mundane. The people, voting with their feet, would leak from Church-controlled to more secular institutions. The Bishops feared that this would diminish their power and the doctors feared that it would diminish their purse. Of course, not all would defect. There are those whose pretension would not allow them to enter the portals of a public hospital. A great many however would fail to see the sense of paying for that which they could receive *gratis*. This would act to the detriment of private institutions and their medical denizens; to quote the Bishop of Ferns, this would not be 'advantageous', 'to the medical profession'.

Many people would flock to public maternity services, and presumably later to other services, because they were free. The remainder, however were a prize still worth fighting for, and the Church-Medical alliance was not prepared to see these also removed because the public services were manifestly superior. To prevent the emergence of such catastrophic excellence in public health services therefore became a war aim in 1950. This has interesting relevance to the profligate use of advertising to promote private healthcare institutions in modern Ireland.

Medical students have long been taught the list of As, the hanging offences of medical practice for which a doctor could be struck off the Medical Register: abortion, adultery and addiction were in the gold, silver and bronze positions. Next came advertising. While the Irish Medical Council might, even today, look askance at a doctor advertising 'I am the greatest', it has become the norm for private hospitals to promote themselves in this way. Thus, amongst other examples, the emergence of the patient-orientated National Cancer Control Programme produced integrated units which were demonstrably superior (with regard to what we are calling scientific or deep excellence) to the improvisations available privately, which were spared the intrusions of HIQUA. The result has been a rash of advertising – we are the greatest. Again threatened by the emergence of excellence in public sector medicine, those elements who in 1950 had sought their salvation through the power of the Hierarchy now resorted instead, in post-God Ireland, to a very different Church, the Church of Madison Avenue – advertising.

23

THE LEGACY

There is little doubt that the future development of the Irish Health service was, in its direction (or perhaps lack of direction) and ideology, determined by the outcome of the Mother and Child conspiracy of 1950.

The Minister for Health of the day, Dr Noël Browne, was in tune with the prevailing *zeitgeist* in health services in Northern Europe and in Great Britain in particular. It is likely that, if he had been permitted to give the population a taste of universal services – what the Bishop of Ferns called 'totalitarian' – it would have whetted the appetite for more. The proposed scheme had universal application only to a particular segment of the population – mothers, and children up to the age of sixteen years. Within that considerable segment, however, everybody, regardless of income, would be entitled to free service. With the public's appetite awakened, the omens for advancement towards a fully integrated comprehensive health service would have been favourable indeed.

In 1950 it would have been cheap enough to institute such a service. Medical science had not yet become the voracious monster that it is today. Specialists were few and generalists reigned. With the exception of managing the infectious diseases, there was not a lot that could be done. One got cataracts and, like John Milton, one went blind. A great many got arthritis of the weight bearing joints and limped painfully or sat by the fire, their demise accelerated by inactivity. There had been little fundamental advance in the treatment of heart disease since the discovery of digitalis in 1785.[182] Money-burning intensive care units did not exist. There was no transplantation, kidney dialysis, cancer chemotherapy, artificial ventilation and the list goes on to include many further expensive interventions commonplace today, and demanded by a population gorged on expectation and entitlement.

The Minister for Finance, and through him ironically the Minister for Health, was the beneficiary of the widespread consumption of tobacco with its attendant revenue raising and life shortening powers. The actuarial nightmare of longevity had not reared its head. Dying was cheap, mostly took place outside of hospitals and was more the business of priests than doctors. Societies at the stage of development at which Ireland was then, are often disproportionately endowed with priests over doctors. Priests, in whatever guise, are cheaper.

Other factors, current in 1950 but long since disappeared, would have oiled the introduction of a properly integrated Irish Health Service.

Ireland then was a country of low expectations: the people, used to little, would have been satisfied with a little more. Doubtless in time expectations would have increased but by then the model would have become embedded and, as happened elsewhere, there would be no going back. Woe betide any future Minister tempted to take back what had been given. He would, doubtless, reflect carefully on the fate of Ernest Blythe.[183] When the Minister giveth he is rewarded with many votes. When, however, he taketh away he is courting electoral oblivion.

The labour market of 1950 was ideal for the initiation of such a comprehensive health project: this has changed utterly. In modern health services the cost of labour is nightmarish to the extent that in hospitals up to 70 per cent of all money available goes on salaries.[184] The more specialised the operative and the more he or she accumulates additional qualifications, vacuous or substantial, the more the salary increases – with no measured increase in productivity. In 1950, the Minister, if he had been allowed to embark on a comprehensive integrated health service, would have encountered little of this. Specialists, even among doctors, were few and among other grades scarcely existent. Labour was cheap and abundant. Hospitals were ruled by the august Matron – she is now replaced by a monstrous regiment and sorely missed. In this benign milieu the Minister for Health, if not sabotaged, could have advanced his project to popular acclaim and at manageable cost.

In 1950, furthermore, the trade unions, with the exception of the doctor's union, would have been on the Minister's side in his efforts to introduce change. Later Ministers for Health, in contrast, seem to have the greatest difficulty coexisting with the latter day workers representatives. Healthcare workers, ironically predominantly female, are represented by a hirsute clone of decidedly Napoleonic tendency. These latter have a legion of journalists hanging on their every drearily predictable word. Thus the Minister of 1950 would have had the support of the unions in introducing epoch making change, while his modern counterparts meet a barrage of objections on any attempt to introduce even the merest departure from the *status quo*. The trade union soil, fertile to change in 1950, has become barren.

In the pre-industrial Ireland of 1950, employing people was a simple process. There was a rate for a job with little overtime. Professionalism, much touted in the modern era where it is more a concept than a reality, reigned. Doctors, nurses and other grades discharged their duties with little expectation of extra money regardless of hours. The Minister for Health could thus budget with precision. All grades in the Health Service, not least doctors, over the years became the recipients of a Byzantine plethora of extra payments and allowances as a reward for discharging what in 1950 would have been regarded as their professional duties. As an example of this it emerged in 2013 – and then only as a result of severe health budget cuts – that management in Voluntary Hospitals were the recipients of no less than thirty-six allowances and extra payments.[185]

In his efforts to introduce an integrated health service in 1950, the Minister for Health would have encountered none of the regulatory overkill or litigious rapacity of the modern epoch. The modest amount of money that he had, he could spend on patients. Medical litigation was negligible and a doctor could insure himself against it, as this writer did, for three pounds per annum. The unnecessary, extravagant, morale sapping show trials[186] of medical professionals, commonplace today, scarcely existed. The Minister, at that time, could rely on the professionalism of the Matron and her nurses, and indeed often the nuns, to keep the hospital clean. Today this has to be enforced by that strange spawn of Celtic Tiger extravagance, HIQUA. Highly paid HIQUA inspectors arrive like the wrath of God to critique the hygiene of wards and much else – fair enough the citizen might think. But the citizen is not made aware that, in many instances, these 'inspectors' are senior staff previously responsible for such wards. Re-inventing themselves – the expression 'gone to HIQUA' gained considerable currency – they apply themselves at great expense and with the zeal of the reformed, to reversing the decrepitude over which they had previously presided.

THE VHI AND RUBBING SHOULDERS

The Irish Statute Book has, as its first enactment of 1957, The Voluntary Health Insurance Act. The organisation to which this gave effect became known thereafter, mostly but not universally with affection, as the VHI. Notwithstanding that the organisation has been a worthy performer and has become part of the national fabric, its founding laid down an ideological marker for the future direction of healthcare delivery in Ireland.

It is worthy of note that between the Mother and Child debacle of 1951 and the VHI Act of 1957, a Fianna Fáil Government under de Valera had come and gone. By 1957 the incumbent of 1950, John A. Costello, having for the second time struggled with his reluctance and lost, was back in the Taoiseach's office.

How the Archbishop of Dublin, John Charles McQuaid, must have rejoiced at the second coming of the reluctant one. Following the unconditional surrender of State to Church in 1951, the Archbishop had been known to write:[187]

> That the clash should have come in this particular form and under this Government, with Mr Costello at its head, is a very happy success for the Church.'

It is clear from this that the Archbishop welcomed the 'clash' as a providential instrument with which to smite nascent secular tendencies and to consolidate the theocracy. It is less than flattering to Mr Costello who he clearly considered to be a pushover. There is the clear message that he would have expected the more Machiavellian de Valera to be less docile. The point is redundant, however, because de Valera would likely have slithered away from the confrontation as he had done oft times before.

With the Archbishop's man back in the Taoiseach's office (1954), plans could now proceed for what His Grace had earlier called 'a sane health service'. Furthermore, the Department of Health was now in what the Archbishop must surely have considered to be a safe pair of hands. Dr Tom O'Higgins, bred in the purple of Fine Gael, would be just the man to advance the health service in a direction which the Archbishop considered 'sane'. Having allowed, in his first Government, a naïve enthusiast to blunder unprotected into the hard hat area of 'Health', only to get clobbered by the Bishops, the Taoiseach, wiser in his second coming, consigned the portfolio to an unquestionably 'sane' man and one of sound conservative outlook. The odious threat of 'no doctor's bills', after a turbulent gestation of eighteen trimesters, was finally stillborn.

From his correspondence we have a clear idea of the Archbishop's blueprint for the future development of the health service. Such development must incorporate the virtues of 'initiative' and 'self reliance'. These twin virtues, so admirable in the individual, may not however be equally so when adopted as the doctrinaire *modus operandi* of the State. The 'rights of private medical practitioners' – such an incongruous preoccupation of the Hierarchy throughout the Mother and Child controversy – should also be protected in any new structures. Most particularly important was that the better off should not have to endure 'a heavy tax' when they might have no 'desire to use the facilities provided'. Interpreted in its least Christian light, this might be taken to mean that the rich would be required, not only to pay for the poor but to rub shoulders with them as well in 'the facilities provided'.

There would be little rubbing of shoulders in the health service ordained by John Charles McQuaid.

The essential thrust of healthcare policy is decided by Governments – the matter is primarily political rather than scientific. The British Government under The National Health Service Act, 1946 (implemented in 1948) consolidated all medical institutions into the new all-embracing national system. Part 1, section 1 of the Act stated specifically the following: 'The services so provided shall be free of charge.'

It is clear that the Irish Minister for Health of 1950, Dr Noël Browne, with his manifesto of 'no doctor's bills' was intent on a similar course of which the Mother and Child Scheme was merely to be the opening shot.

Anathema though the Archbishop and his medical abettors might have found the 'no doctor's bills' proclamation, there was something even more odious in the British legislation, something even the remotest possibility of which would have rendered His Grace apoplectic. This radical step, taken by the British, was entirely necessary to the introduction of an integrated, comprehensive and fair system. Likewise, failure to take this step in Ireland made fragmentation, duplication, dysfunction, political jobbery, and the triumph of sectional interests inevitable.

Part 11, 6(1) of the British National Health Service Act was headed by the ominous words: 'Transfer of hospitals to the Minister.'

In its text the section stated the following:

> Subject to the provisions of this Act, there shall, on the appointed day, be transferred and vest in the Minister by virtue of this Act all interests in or attaching to premises forming part of a voluntary hospital or used for the purpose of a voluntary hospital.

The 'Mother of Parliaments' knew that it would be impossible to knock the new Government Health Service into any kind of decent shape without owning and fully controlling the hospitals. Therein lay the rub in 1950. In Ireland the hospitals were, in almost all important instances, owned by the Church and the Church was, *de facto*, controlled by the Archbishop of Dublin. He would, with some justification, have considered 'transfer of hospitals to the Minister' as confiscation. The confiscations of the Reformation had deprived John Charles McQuaid of his cathedral. He was not about to allow the Minister's 'reformation' of the Health Service to deprive him of his hospitals.

Yet there was need of a revenue stream to run the hospitals. In Britain this revenue stream was derived from taxation, but the Archbishop, a doctrinaire conservative, had objected to 'a heavy tax for the purpose'. It was not so much that he wished to spare the citizens from the attentions of the Revenue Commissioners, but rather that with public funding would come loss of control of his fief. A new stream of revenue must therefore be devised and it must be independent of Government – it must be private.

To devise a structure to serve this purpose which would, at the same time, meet all the prescriptive requirements of His Grace, required some genius. Regular insurance companies in the Ireland of 1950 would see little dividend from such an enterprise. The State then – the same State for the officers of which the Archbishop had shown such contempt – must be induced to act as midwife. And now was the time, with Mr Costello back in power, to deliver this new infant into the world. Indeed, another 'happy success' beckoned not just for the Church but particularly for the medical profession. Once delivered, however, the newborn health insurance entity must, apart from perfunctory regulatory oversight, assume a near independent existence. It would, enigmatically, be dependent on the State for its existence but independent of the State in its functioning – nice work if you can get it.

The Voluntary Health Insurance Board was to be 'a body corporate', submitting, once a year, its audited accounts to the Minister for Health of the day. Disbursement of the revenue stream was entirely at the discretion of the Board. In the early years and for many decades thereafter the lion's share of this disbursement went precisely where the Archbishop had intended. Indeed, successive Ministers for Health regulated operation of the Act in a manner which hobbled certain public hospitals, while public parts of less secular institutions were allowed to collect every penny.

The Voluntary Health Insurance Act (1957) is admirably concise and adroit in its drafting. Nowhere in any of the twenty-seven sections does the word 'private' appear.

Now the Government had nailed its colours clearly to the mast. A system of healthcare which had shown signs of drifting to the left and towards egalitarianism was sharply jolted to the right by an Act of the Oireachtas. The Archbishop's prescription, as set out in his correspondence, was being administered to the nation by a captive Government and, for good measure, included the 'taxation relief' advocated by the Bishop of Ferns. The new Voluntary Health Insurance was then promoted by a vigorous publicity campaign particularly in cinemas which, although heavily censored, were one of the main communications media of the time. To be fair, the thrust of the advertising was that the VHI was for everybody – a noble, if naïve, objective. Cinemagoers, before escaping into the sanitised peregrinations of Scarlett O'Hara and Rhett Butler[188] or the King of Siam,[189] were first regaled with the VHI jingle. The rhyming couplet went:

> The family safeguard all can afford
> The Voluntary Health Insurance Board.

These observations are not in the least censorious of the VHI *per se*. It has discharged its responsibilities as set out in the Act, and as directed by successive Ministers for Health. Its birth however marked the onset of the Government's schizoid approach to healthcare funding. Regardless of its light touch regulation, the VHI was, after all, and still is owned by the Government. Thus the Government was, thereafter, involved in raising revenue for healthcare through two chalk and cheese organisations, both of which it owned – the Revenue Commissioners and the Voluntary Health Insurance Board. Precisely how the Government of 1957 believed this would develop is not easy to divine. It is likely, however, that it acted in good faith but with no small naïveté. A less charitable interpretation would be that they recognised that a duality of funding would, inevitably, result in a duality of service, but were comfortable with this. This duality has resulted in what, in their disgruntlement, the people now call a 'two tier system'.

There is little doubt that the Archbishop of Dublin was exceedingly comfortable with the birth of the VHI; his fingerprints are all over it as they were with the Constitution. Throughout the Mother and Child controversy he had insisted that the burden of healthcare should be carried by 'voluntary' institutions, and now this very word appeared in the title of the new entity – another 'happy success' for His Grace. His prescription for the health service became Government policy and was now enshrined in law. His Grace's anxiety about Ministerial 'resort to statutory instruments', which had so exercised him during the Mother and Child affair, had magically dissipated.

It was not long, however, before it became clear that Voluntary Health Insurance was not something that 'all can afford'. Nor was it long before those who made the commendable effort to pay the premium – 85,000 subscribed in the first three years – began, with every justification, to expect something over and above that which was made available to those dismissed by the Hierarchy as the 'necessitous 10 per cent'. This was entirely understandable but it was equally predictable. The die was now cast, however. With Government and Episcopal sanction, those seeking hospital care in the future would be triaged as much by their means as by their pathology.

It is entirely proper that private medical institutions should, in a free market, exist and if they can prosper, good luck to them: they often extract efficiencies not seen in the public sector. It should not, however, be the business of Government in a Republic to acquiesce in, and indeed own, structures the inevitable consequence of which is to triage patients according to their money rather than their pathology. Since 1957, the consequence of the Archbishop's prescription has inevitably and increasingly resulted in those endowed with 'initiative' and 'self reliance' (his words) having 'no desire to use the facilities provided' (again his words), as a public service for the generality of the citizens. The health service which has emerged is not perceived as fair and does not contribute to social cohesion – it does not encourage the rubbing of shoulders.

Scientific Advance and Economic Retreat

For a time the hybrid health system worked reasonably. The Government, in an era when it was cheap to do so, could afford to provide acceptable services for 'the necessitous'. Likewise, those of 'initiative' and 'self reliance' were happy in their apartheid comforts. The hybrid system became normalised. Perhaps the Archbishop, with two millennia of institutional experience behind him, had been right after all!

Alas not so. Two dynamics rained on the parade: scientific advance and economic retreat.

Many of the great advances in medicine up to 1950 had been microbiological and inexpensive enough to implement. The inside of the cell, theretofore almost a no go area, began to give up its secrets, raising the possibility of designer drugs.

Perhaps the first significant blow was struck in 1964 with the discovery of the heart drug Propranolol.[190] Digitalis, cheap and king of the cardiac castle since 1785, was unceremoniously dumped into history. Propranolol immediately became the biggest selling drug – and the most lucrative. It became the business of stockbrokers as much as doctors. The financial community, which has always found the language of Shakespeare inadequate to express its thoughts, required a new lexicon. Enter the 'blockbuster drug'. These latter drugs are produced, under strict patent, by a species of company which has come to be known (or demonised[191]), to the dubious improvement of the English language, as 'Big Pharma'. In order to join the pantheon of blockbusters, a drug must achieve sales of one billion dollars per annum. Propranolol, although a worthy candidate, in simpler economic times, never joined the Gods.

A decade later, however, the same Scottish genius, James Black, who had discovered Propranolol struck again with the ulcer drug Cimetidine – the first blockbuster drug had arrived and prospered for decades even eventually making generic drug makers rich.[192] Cimetidine did something unusual in medicine: it paid for itself by beginning the process of abolishing ulcer surgery. Rather than costing them a fortune, funding agencies, private and public, were saving money. This benevolence of Big Pharma would not last.

Big Pharma became the hot investment topic. Money managers, who scarcely knew what a molecule was, waxed lyrical about side-chains. But the drugs worked, the patients clamoured and the funders paid. Preventative mass medication became the vogue. The Irish Government provided the drugs free for 'the necessitous' and subsidised for the better off – a double whammy.

The cholesterol lowering drug Atorvastatin (Lipitor) was launched in 1996 and did not come off patent until 2011. Used for mass medication, it achieved annual sales of twelve billion dollars worldwide. A plethora of other blockbusters arrived. In 2011 Americans spent $320 billion on the top 20 drugs alone.[193] Even Uncle Sam was showing the strain of this: lesser countries, including Ireland, were left for dead. During this orgy, Big Pharma, protected by patents, could get away with predatory pricing. The unflattering term 'Bad Pharma' began to appear. In dealing with predatory pricing, health funders of the time, public and private, were a poor match for the marketing acumen of Big Pharma.

In step with the development of blockbuster drugs, all branches of medicine advanced expensively into the realm of the unaffordable. Surgeries, previously unimaginable, advanced apace across the full spectrum. Almost everything became replaceable or transplantable. Advances in materials and engineering brought profits from medical devices and hardware into the blockbuster category. Business conspired to make most of these devices disposable at the expense of budgets and the environment.[194] Medicine became phenomenally successful but prohibitively expensive. Healthcare expenditure in the United States reached 18 per cent of Gross Domestic Product; in Ireland it got to 9 per cent.

Drug and equipment budgets ran amok and became parasitic on the overall system, but particularly on the public system dealing with the less well off. Private institutions could cover the increased cost by raising insurance premia. Furthermore, when the private patient was discharged back into the community from the apartheid institution, his drugs were heavily subsidised from the public purse to the further detriment of the public service, which began to show cracks.

These cracks in the public healthcare provision are greatly exacerbated by the vagaries of the economic cycle. Although often completely predictable, cyclical economic downturns seem to come as a complete surprise to the Irish citizens and their leaders. Time and again ability to fund the public health system had been undermined by such shocks, much to the detriment of its reputation.

The more the public system cracked, the more people, understandably, subscribed to private health insurance. This enabled them to triage themselves away from (in the Archbishop's words) 'the facilities provided' for the common run of citizens. Either by Government design or incompetence, a new term was added to the lexicon – the 'two tier system' had arrived and put down deep roots. These roots had their origin in the conspiracy of 1951 and the legislation of 1957 – the destruction of Noël Browne and the Voluntary Health Insurance Act respectively.

The more impossibly expensive medicine became the more fissures appeared in the public system to the detriment of its reputation. This added to the allure of the private system. John Charles McQuaid and his disciples would not have been surprised by any of this: private good, public bad. But the two teams, public and private, competing in the dysfunctional Irish healthcare system never played on a level pitch.

FICTION OF A FREE MARKET

The received wisdom that private medicine in Ireland is independently funding itself in a free market is a fiction.

Apart from the already mentioned tax relief on health insurance premia and community drug subsidies, there is a raft of additional fiscal perversions and distortions of the free market in which successive Governments have acquiesced, in the spirit of the McQuaid blueprint of 1950. This works, predominantly, to the benefit of the middle classes who, for much routine work, triage themselves to private institutions, but for complex and expensive conditions, particularly those of a chronic nature, resort to the public system, as has been made their right.

Emergency medicine, emergency surgery and trauma are cases in point. Most private hospitals in Ireland are allowed to spare themselves the expense and trouble of maintaining and staffing a full emergency department and none does so for twenty-four hours[195] – there is no money in it. In this regard the public hospitals do the heavy lifting – and spending. Public secular hospitals, while taking the hit for expensive work, and all of obstetrics and extremely expensive neonatology, are prevented from structuring themselves as enterprises to compete for less exacting elements of the service from which they could make a profit.

The ambulance, carrying the case that will break the bank, races past the private hospital to deposit him in the public emergency department. The patient, perhaps being well heeled, may have no desire to find himself in such a proletarian place or as the Archbishop put it, 'to avail of the facilities provided'. There is, however, no place else for him to go. The cherry pickers do not want him.

Even in the United States, where the healthcare system is scarcely known for its altruism, the Government has stepped in to stop this cherry picking abuse. Hospitals are compelled by law[196] to maintain emergency departments and look after the 'necessitous' at considerable expense. The law giving effect to this compulsion, the Emergency Treatment and Labour Law (EMTLA), has entered the uninhibited popular American lexicon as 'the patient anti-dumping law'. In the United States in 2004, 55 per cent of such EMTALA expenditures, amounting to 40.7 billion dollars, went unpaid for in private hospitals which had to carry the cost – a subsidy from private to public amounting to 6 per cent of total hospital spending. The Irish cherry pickers are spared the shoulder rubbing which this would involve. To compound the iniquity, the patient who has been private all his life may, when in emergency, or smitten by expensive to treat pathology, declare himself 'public' and pay almost nothing. And, to make matters worse, because of the urgency of his case he shoulders aside the normal clientele of the public hospital whose operation for gallstones or hernia or joint replacement is cancelled to the further detriment of the institution's reputation. Public bad: private good. And all of this in addition to the 'dumping' of the entirety of obstetrics on the public sector while its associated gynaecology remains suitable for cherry picking.

In the twenty-first century there has been a proliferation of private hospitals of scarcely critical mass in Ireland. These are, *de facto*, massively subsidised by the public purse. For them, the much touted free market means they are free to cherry pick, while dumping resource-intensive patients on the public system. Thus as the public hospital system struggles with its Sisyphean labours, the cleavage between those of 'initiative' and 'self reliance', and the 'necessitous' widens, to the detriment of social cohesion and national morale.

When a private hospital implants expensive prosthetic items, it charges for the materials, and rightly so – indeed, by charging 'corkage', it may make a profit on the item. All consumable items are totted up and reimbursed, again rightly so (even if a global figure is negotiated for the procedure, such items are taken into account in arriving at that figure). The secular public hospital, on the other hand, is forbidden to charge private patients for such materials by Ministerial decree – the playing field between public and private is tilted. In good times this has little effect. Come economic retreat, however, implants on the public side, for example joint replacements, get rationed, the service contracts and the 'necessitous' citizen limps on.

It is commonplace for patients in private facilities, who need, for example, kidney dialysis, to be transferred to the public system. While this makes sense, particularly for the patient, the private system is spared the vast investment in infrastructure required to provide such facilities. Likewise, certain private facilities undertake lucrative cardiac catheterisations without the backup of cardiac surgery on site if things go wrong. This sub-optimal arrangement works only because it is backed up by the public system. The public system is carrying the risk for the private – and risk, as we have already discussed, is expensive.

While no actuarial audit of this subsidy exists, it is clear that, *de facto*, resources are moving from left (public) to right (private). In the United States, by contrast, the Government, using the EMTALA Act, is happy to acquiesce in the shunting of resources, to the extent of the 6 per cent already discussed, from right to left.

Hybrid System and Economic Retreat

The greatest resource in any healthcare system is personnel: salaries, after all, make up the greater part of expenditure (up to 70 per cent in hospitals). Education, training, experience and skill are of the essence. It is the public service, almost exclusively – and very expensively – which is responsible for the inculcation of these attributes. Specialist senior doctors' salaries and pensions are a huge burden on the public system: most private hospitals pay none. With regard to consultant doctor staffing, private hospitals pull a master stroke. They extend privileges to a great many public hospital consultant employees at no cost and much profit. The Department of Health, true to the McQuaid doctrine of 1950, acquiesces in, and indeed encourages this. Foreign specialists, who visit our institutions, are uncomprehending of these arrangements.

Consultant doctors in the public service work to a bewildering array of contracts which might have been concocted by Gilbert and Sullivan. Many, finding themselves inadequately resourced on the public side during times of economic retreat, are driven, not always reluctantly, to work increasingly in private hospitals, thus to provide skills which might otherwise not be available there, and so to prop up the hybrid system.

An independent observer might expect a large differential in salary between a consultant doctor who works only in the public hospital and a colleague who works there and also works (perhaps extensively) in a private hospital. The differential, however, in order to support the hybrid system, has been kept derisory. Under this hybrid system, doctors' traditional Hippocratic advocacy for good public services has tended to atrophy. This does the profession little credit. Instead of fighting for resources on the public side, they surrender to a convenient despair and decamp to prop up private institutions – but remain permanent and pensionable on the public side.

Ireland is a medical cherry pickers' paradise.

Investors can make money out of private hospital medicine only if they are allowed to cherry pick. In Ireland, venture capitalists ranging from property developers to cattle dealers to entrepreneurial doctors have come to the trough. The involvement of the latter is particularly dubious. In the United States, the Government, with an alacrity not to be expected any time soon from the Irish Government or the Irish Medical Council, has banned doctors from owning or investing in hospitals.[197] The doctors in the United States were, in effect, scandalously referring to themselves and to their diagnostic departments. This creaming off of lucrative straightforward cases roused the reputable hospital sector to fury – and to lobby. The Patient Protection and Affordable Care Act (2010), known colloquially as 'Obamacare', and greeted with little affection by the medical establishment, prohibits physician investment in hospitals.

The American government recognised that the backbone of the hospital system was being eroded by cherry picking and patient dumping, an expression which we are too delicate in Ireland to use.

Yet the Irish Government encourages cherry picking at every turn. A buckshot of new private 'hospitals', sometimes shoe-horned into redundant Celtic Tiger era buildings, and to date exempted from the demanding inspections of HIQUA, is lauded as progress when, in fact, it is retrograde. Two generations of painful hospital rationalisation is being negated by *laissez faire* and lack of an integrated policy.

CONCLUSION

Thus the Health Service which the Irish people have inherited is fragmented and not fit for purpose: it is the legacy of the Archbishop's victory of 1951. Until all hospitals are subsumed into some kind of unitary integrated system – public, private or, more likely, with elements of both – chaos will endure. Although the middle classes are not entirely spared the effects of medical chaos, it bears most heavily on the less well off – those characterised by the Archbishop of Dublin as 'necessitous' and by the Irish Medical Association as 'indigent'. The discomforts of the 'necessitous' and the 'indigent' perturb politicians altogether less than the lobbying of the middle classes. The lobbying of these latter brought about the containment of the AIDS menace in the United States within a time frame that even the most optimistic did not envisage. In healthcare the meek, contrary to received biblical wisdom, do not inherit the earth. These same articulate educated elements in Ireland are, to a considerable extent, removed from the debate by their better access to services and comforts, often within cherry picking institutions.

The Irish healthcare industry, although of considerable size and containing foci of excellence, does not amount to a system – a system implies integration of the parts. Vested interests, exemplified *par excellence* by John Charles McQuaid, but hardly less by medical organisations, local politicians and lobbyists for scarcely viable hospitals, have contrived to produce not integration but Balkanisation. This has resulted in a service where the outcome is less than the potential sum of the parts. The debacle of 1951 fortified the already ample Voluntary Hospital institutional chauvinism and this has endured. The verbiage of the Archbishop and his associates, for example the President of University College Cork, was condescending in the extreme towards 'State' institutions. As late as 2015 such voluntary institutions, although almost entirely funded by the State, felt it was not the business of the taxpayers' representatives to monitor how they spent that money.[198] In the face of this temerity and institutional chauvinism, politicians appeared to a despairing public to be impotent and pathetic.

While all countries, including Ireland, have a problem funding healthcare, the issue is generally one of resources. The resource problem in Ireland, while undeniable, is compounded by the organisational structures that have been inherited.

The McQuaid effect has proven more durable in hospitals than in churches – a final irony.

Appendix I

LETTER FROM BISHOP OF FERNS TO THE TAOISEACH

10 October 1950

Dear Taoiseach,

The Archbishops and Bishops of Ireland, at their meeting on October 10th, had under consideration the proposals for Mother and Child health service and other kindred medical services. They recognise that these proposals are motivated by a sincere desire to improve the public health, but they feel bound by their office to consider whether the proposals are in accordance with Catholic moral teaching.

In their opinion the powers taken by the State in the proposed Mother and Child Health service are in direct opposition to the rights of the family and of the individual and are liable to very great abuse. Their character is such that no assurance that they would be used in moderation could justify their enactment. If adopted in law they would constitute a ready-made instrument for future totalitarian aggression.

The right to provide for the health of children belongs to parents not to the State. The State has the right to intervene only in a subsidiary capacity, to supplement, not to supplant.

It may help indigent or neglectful parents; it may not deprive 90 per cent of parents of their rights because of 10 per cent necessitous or negligent parents.

It is not sound social policy to impose a state medical service on the whole community on the pretext of relieving the necessitous 10 per cent from the so-called indignity of the means test.

The right to provide for the physical education of children belongs to the family and not to the State. Experience has shown that physical or health education is closely interwoven with important moral questions on which the Catholic Church had definite teaching.

Education in regard to motherhood includes instruction in regard to sex relations, chastity and marriage. The State has no competence to give instruction in such matters. we regard with the greatest apprehension the proposal to give to local medical officers the right to tell Catholic girls and women how they should behave in regard to this sphere of conduct at once so delicate and sacred.

Gynaecological care may be, and in some countries is interpreted to include provision for birth limitation and abortion. We have no guarantee that State officials will respect Catholic principles in regard to these matters. Doctors trained in institutions in which we have no confidence may be appointed as medical officers under the proposed services may give gynaecological care not in accordance with Catholic principles.

The proposed service also destroys the confidential relations between doctor and patient and regards all cases of illness as matter for public records and research without regard to the individual's right to privacy.

The elimination of private medical practitioners by a State-paid service has not been shown to be necessary or even advantageous to the patient, the public in general or the medical profession.

The Bishops are most favourable to measures which would benefit public health, but they consider that instead of imposing a costly bureaucratic scheme of nationalised medical advice the State might well consider the advisability of providing the maternity hospitals and other institutional facilities which are at present lacking and should give adequate maternity benefits and taxation relief for large families.

The Bishops desire that your Government should give careful consideration to the dangers inherent in the present proposals before they are adopted by the Government for legislative enactment and, therefore they feel it their duty to submit their views on this subject to you privately and at the earliest opportunity, since they regard the issues involved as of the greatest moral and religious importance.

I remain, dear Taoiseach

Yours very sincerely,

(Sgd.) James Staunton,

Bishop of Ferns,

Secretary to the Hierarchy.

Appendix 2

LETTER FROM TAOISEACH TO BISHOP OF FERNS

28 March 1951

My Lord Bishop,

I beg to enclose a memorandum of observations of the Minister for Health on various matters relating to the Mother and Child Scheme referred to in a letter dated the 10th October 1950 addressed to me by Your Lordship as Secretary to the Hierarchy. May I be allowed to state that since the receipt by me from His Grace of Dublin of Their Lordships' letter my colleagues and I have given anxious consideration to the objections made by the Hierarchy to the scheme advocated by the Minister for Health. His Grace of Dublin has on many occasions seen me in the interval and kindly agreed to inform the standing committee that the Government would readily and immediately acquiesce in a decision of the Hierarchy concerning faith and morals. If I have not answered earlier and in detail the letter of the Hierarchy I trust that it will be understood that both His Grace of Dublin and I believed it to be much more advantageous in the special circumstances of the case to await developments. Within recent weeks the publication by the Minister for Health of a brochure explaining his scheme called forth from His Grace of Dublin an immediate reply in which His Grace re-iterated each and every objection already made by him to the Scheme.

After an interview with His Grace in which the Minister had been again warned of His Grace's objections and had himself asked for an early decision of the Hierarchy the Minister for Health forwarded to me the enclosed memorandum.

His Grace of Dublin has kept me accurately informed of these latter circumstances and has kindly agreed to request Your Lordship as the Most Reverend Secretary to include the Minister's observations on the agenda of the forthcoming meeting of the Hierarchy.

John A Costello, Taoiseach.

Notes

1. Otto von Bismarck Chancellor and unifier of modern Germany (1815-1898). Early European advocate of social welfare and health insurance. Lloyd George's British Health Insurance Act, 1911 was based on Bismarck's thinking, a fact rarely acknowledged. Bismarck saw such benefits as a device to placate the masses and garner votes, hence – 'Politics is the art of the possible'.

2. Tithe. One-tenth of one's income contributed to a religious organisation. Much resented in Ireland as majority Catholics had to support minority Protestant Church. Abolished as result of 'The Tithe War', 1830-1836.

3. American Republican Party millionaire supporter Tom Perkins said on CNN Money in February 2014 that rich people (who pay more taxes) should have more votes than others who pay less.

4. 'The Patient Protection and Affordable Care Act'. United States Federal Statute. 2012. Known colloquially as 'Obamacare'.

5. 'Small Government'. Associated with Ronald Reagan Presidency (1980-1988) now incarnated in the right wing 'Tea Party' faction.

6. Louis Pasteur (1822-1895). French. Pioneer microbiologist said of his discoveries, 'Luck favours the prepared mind'.

7. Joseph Lister (1827-1912). British. Applied modern aseptic techniques in surgery at Glasgow Royal Infirmary.

8. Ignaz Semmelweis (1818-1865). Hungarian. Early advocate of hand washing to minimise infection. Scorned by sceptical medical establishment of his time.

9. Robert Koch (1843-1905). German. Identified bacterium which causes tuberculosis. Nobel Prize, 1905.

10. Validating a hypothesis by reproducible scientific experiment or measurement. The basis of modern 'Evidence Based Medicine'.

11. O'Brien, E. The Charitable Infirmary, Jervis Street: Chronology of a Voluntary Hospital. J. Irish Colleges of Physicians and Surgeons, (1984).13:56-66. Charitable Infirmary Jervis St (1718), extinct. Dr

Steevens Hospital, 1720, extinct. North Charitable Infirmary, Cork (1744), extinct. Mercers Hospital, 1745, extinct. Rotunda Hospital, 1745, extant. Meath Hospital, 1753, extinct. South Charitable Infirmary, Cork (1761) extant. Waterford County and City Infirmary (1785), extinct. Barrington's Hospital, Limerick (1829), extant (now private) etc.

12. Notably Paul Cullen (1803-1878). Cardinal Archbishop of Dublin. Of the 'strong farmer' class. His father owned 700 acres of prime Kildare.

13. Notably St Vincent's, Dublin (1834). Mercy, Cork (1857). Mater, Dublin (1861). Mater Infirmorum, Belfast, 1883.

14. Republic of Ireland Act (1948). Severed connection with the crown.

15. *Caritas.* Latin for charity.

16. Dives and Lazarus: Luke 16: 19-31.

17. Matthew 26:11.

18. The Charities Act 2009 is the latest of many iterations. It defines a 'charitable purpose' as including along with much else, the 'advancement of religion'.

19. 'Political bishops'. Attributed in the Irish context to Henry Grattan (1746-1820). Used by Noël Browne to deride his clerical adversaries. He referred to McQuaid as 'the chief political Bishop'. Cooney, John. *John Charles McQuaid: Ruler of Catholic Ireland.* Dublin: O'Brien Press, 2003, p. 264.

20. The Irish Meteorological Service cooperated fully with the Allies. A break in the foul weather at Belmullet was telegraphed by Paddy Sweeney to Allied HQ enabling Eisenhower to proceed with the Normandy landings. *Southern Ireland and the Liberation of France*: Gerald Morgan and Gavin Hughes. Peter Lang A G, Berne, 2011, p. 206.

21. *Punch.* Racist London periodical. 'The missing link'. 1862. Referring to 'the Irish Yahoo', 'It is moreover a climbing animal and may sometimes be seen ascending a ladder with a hod of bricks'.

22. Donovan. Song. *Universal Soldier.* 1964. 'He's the one who gives his body as a weapon of the war'.

23. John B. Keane (1928-2002). Play. *Many Young Men of Twenty.* (1961). Lampooned emigration and hypocrisy.

24. Orphan Annie. American cartoon character with empty eyes. Appearance used to describe certain cells in thyroid cancer.

25. Unflattering moniker for England implying capacity for duplicity. Unsurprisingly, much resorted to by the French in matters of

international diplomacy. Possibly related to the white (Alba) cliffs of Dover, visible from France.

26. Half a million out of a population of 3 million emigrated in the 1950s. Only Ireland and East Germany, in Europe, suffered population decline in that decade. Daly, Mary. *Slow failure, population decline and independent Ireland: 1920-1973*. Wisconsin University Press, 2006, p. 58.

27. A bone deforming disease of malnutrition and poverty prevented by calcium (abundant in milk) and exposure to sun. Rickets was still commonplace during the author's undergraduate years of the 1960s.

28. 'Mixed Bathing' was amongst the many *bêtes noires* of the Bishop of Galway, Michael Browne (1895-1980).

29. Barrington, Ruth. *Health Medicine and Politics in Ireland 1900-1970*. Dublin: Institute of Public Administration, 1987, p. 129. Barrington characterises the attitude of successive early Irish Governments to tuberculosis as 'despair'. The word might equally describe the Government attitude to the entire Health Service at this time of writing.

30. Two hundred cases of poliomyelitis were reported to the Irish Department of Health in 1950.

31. The preposterous figure of surgeon Sir Lancelot Spratt (James Robertson Justice) endures from this epoch. British film comedy, 'Doctor in the House', 1954.

32. The Department of Health was then accommodated in the splendour of Gandon's Custom House.

33. Letter from Hierarchy to Taoiseach 10 October 1950. National Archives TSCH/3/514997A

34. Roberts, Geoffrey. *Stalin's Wars*. Yale University Press, 2007. In 1990 Margaret Thatcher also used this expression regarding another Russian leader, Mikhail Gorbachev.

35. The Russians exploded their atomic bomb in August 1949 and the Americans dubbed it Joe-1 (after Josef Stalin who was no longer good old Uncle Joe). Klaus Fuchs, an émigré German mathematician, who had worked on the Manhattan Project, was morally concerned about American monopoly of the Atomic Bomb. Ideologically motivated, he gave the secrets to the Russians. He was arrested in London in January 1950 and immediately admitted everything. Sentenced to 15 years, he served eight. He got off lighter than Julius and Ethel Rosenberg, arrested in 1950 and vindictively executed by the Eisenhower administration in 1953.

36. Although discredited (the Tydings Committee called his allegations, which started in February 1950, 'a fraud and a hoax') McCarthy was

given a 'Solemn Pontifical Requiem Mass' in Washington Cathedral. He died of alcoholic liver disease.

37. McCarthy along with 'The House Un-American Activities Committee' (of which McCarthy was not a member), in a communist witch-hunt, persecuted intellectuals and drove many out. McQuaid's (slightly more subtle) policies were likewise aimed at the intellectual cleansing of Ireland.

38. McQuaid letter to Taoiseach 5 April 1951. National Archives, TSCH/3/514997A

39. Hoover's blackmailing depravity is well described throughout Anthony Summers' book *Official and Confidential: The Secret Life of J. Edgar Hoover*. New York: GP Putnam Sons, 1993.

40. Cooney, John. *John Charles McQuaid: Ruler of Catholic Ireland*. Dublin: O'Brien Press, 2003, pp. 228-230. Catholic Information Bureau.

41. McQuaid and Hoover employed similar methods, were mutual admirers and corresponded. Letter Hoover to McQuaid. 1958. Dublin Diocesan Archive AB8/B/XVIII.

42. Greene, Graham. *Our Man in Havana*. London: Heineman, 1958. Made into British film comedy. 1959. Vacuum cleaner salesman (Alec Guinness) recruited by British Intelligence fabricated rocket blueprints from vacuum cleaner parts to dupe his 'control' in London to continue his payment.

43. British film comedy. 1959. (Peter Sellers). Typical of the turmoil of industrial life in the fifties decade.

44. Pinkerton Detective Agency supplied 'muscle' to bosses to break up strikes, notably against the secret Irish 'Molly McGuires'.

45. Browne resigned in April 1951 before Burgess and McLean defected in May. What more convenient and timely evidence could McQuaid and the IMA have hoped for to justify their actions?

46. The British 'Report of the Inter-Departmental Committee on Social Insurance and Allied Services', 1942, described 'The Five Great Evils' as Squalor, Ignorance, Want, Idleness and Disease.

47. American right wing advocacy group named after Baptist missionary/ spy killed by Chinese Communists in 1945. Opposed to Civil Rights Act, 1964 as well as to government intervention and wealth redistribution.

48. Barnett, Corelli. *The Audit of War*. London: Pan, 2001, p. 29.

49. McQuaid letter to Taoiseach 5 April 1951. National Archives, TSCH/3/514997A

50. Matthew 2:16. Fearing loss of his throne to the newborn prophesised

'King of the Jews', Herod (the Great) ordered the killing of all male infants.

51. Luke 3:11

52. Hippocrates. Greek (c. 460 -370 BC). Father of medicine.

53. A slight often attributed incorrectly to Napoleon but first used by Adam Smith in *The Wealth of Nations* (1776).

54. Verbatim from *Irish Medical Association Proposal for a Voluntary Contributory State-Aided Medical Scheme*. 1951. Dublin Diocesan Archive L/77/1/1, p. 5.

55. Named after Roman general Quintus Fabius Maximus the Cunctator (delayer) who rather than engage in frontal battle with Hannibal, wore him down with guerrilla tactics. The Fabians espoused machination rather than revolution to advance the socialist cause.

56. The Cleveland Clinic, employing doctors on the basis of (albeit generous) salary, repeatedly scores top for heart care in the United States. *US News and World Report*, 2014. Also top for kidney disease. *US News and World Report*, 2015. This method of remuneration is more the norm than the exception in many top flight American hospitals. Such doctors are attracted less by money than by the vibrant scientific environment and organisational structure. These latter are neglected in contemporary Ireland with consequent indifferent recruitment and declining standards.

57. In 1950 the American Medical Association (AMA), following an inspection, excluded Irish medical schools (not Belfast) from recognition. In 1951 The New York Board of Regents requested an inspection and the NUI refused. NUI medical graduates were excluded by New York. In 1953 the AMA visited again and reported 'The Irish programme does not suit American standards'. In 1959 the New York Board of Regents visited again and noted 'remarkable improvement' and reinstated recognition. UCC Archive, UC/PO/1459.

58. Long before it happened in 586 BC, Jeremiah prophesied the destruction of Jerusalem by the Babylonian Nebuchadnezzar: one of many such destructions of the Holy City.

59. Charles Maurice de Talleyrand-Perigord (1754-1838). French aristocrat, Minister, Bishop, diplomat, fixer and legendary survivor.

60. Tammany Hall. Corrupt, largely Irish, New York Democratic Party political machine, dominating New York politics. Founded 1786.

61. Prendergast organisation in Kansas City similar to Tammany. Achieved election of Harry Truman as President (1945-1953).

62. The Good Friday liturgy described the Jews as 'Perfidious'. In the 1920s

the Society of Friends of Israel tried to have this removed, to no avail. It was finally removed by Pope John XXIII (1958-1963).

63. Shakespeare, *The Merchant of Venice*, Shylock, Act 1, Scene 3. 'I will feed fat the ancient grudge I bear him'.

64. Roman Stoic philosopher (4BC-65AD). McQuaid was an avid student of Seneca.

65. The ban was not, in fact, McQuaid's creation. It had been smouldering for decades, but he enforced it with vigour. It was abolished in 1970.

66. The story of a sexually fluent American undergraduate at Trinity, Sebastian Dangerfield. Not published in McQuaid's libido-quenched Ireland. A cult book selling millions of copies and still going strong. Dunleavy, J. P., *The Ginger Man*. Paris: Olympia Press, 1955.

67. Gordon Wilson, following the death of his daughter in the Enniskillen Remembrance Day bombing (1987), displayed exemplary Christian forgiveness.

68. Browne was educated, by scholarship, at the Jesuit Public School, Beaumont College, in Berkshire.

69. Streptomycin, isolated in 1943 by Albert Schatz at Rutgers University, New Jersey. He was cheated of most of the credit, his boss Selman Waksman getting a Nobel Prize.

70. Thomas Jefferson (1743-1826). Author of American Declaration of Independence. He believed there should be 'a wall of separation between Church and State'.

71. The street vendor of the Cork *Evening Echo*, now happily better shod, still promotes his wares at full shout on strategic city corners. Such barefoot misery is well evoked (albeit somewhat earlier) by a Jack B. Yeats painting 'Bachelors Walk'. NGI exhibition, May 2015.

72. Louis XIV of France. 'I am the State'.

73. Orwell, George. *1984*. London: Secker and Warburg, 1949.

74. Huxley, Aldous. *Brave New World*. London: Chatto and Windus, 1932.

75. *Batman*, science fiction movie, 1989. Portrayed urban dystopia.

76. Soon after his inauguration, in a break with tradition, Pope Francis said the Church had been too focussed on certain issues including contraception. It must find 'a new balance'. *USA Today*, September 19, 2013.

77. *Roe v. Wade*. 1973. United States Supreme Court decision legalising abortion.

78. David Steele, British politician responsible for the Abortion Act, 1967.

79. Archbishop Diarmuid Martin, 'We have in fact one of the lowest rates of maternal mortality in the world'. Patsy McGarry, *The Irish Times*. 19-11-2012.

80. Macpherson, G. 1948: a turbulent gestation for the NHS, *BMJ*, 1998 Jan 3; 316 (7124):6.

81. An inversion of the American revolutionary slogan (Ben Franklin). 'No taxation [by the British Parliament] without representation [in that parliament]'.

82. The author, along with a group of Irish surgeons visiting Rome for a conference in the 1980s, was received at the Irish Embassy to the Italian Republic. He asked the question of a member of staff, 'is the Embassy busy'? The reply came, 'by no means: all the action is over at the Vatican'.

83. A reserved sin was one of such gravity that it could not be absolved by the regular priest confessor. It had to be confessed to a Bishop.

84. An authoritative ruling by a learned figure in Islam.

85. Horgan, John. *Noel Browne: Passionate Outsider*. Dublin: Gill and Macmillan, 2000. This aspect of Browne's character is well developed throughout the book.

86. Browne was at pains always to sign with a dieresis (Noël) rather than the less exotic Noel which, perish the thought, might be pronounced Nole. While we can accommodate him in this regard here, the typewriters of his Department in 1950 appear to have lacked this facility.

87. Clann na Poblachta, led by Sean McBride, contributed 10 seats to a kaleidoscopic coalition Government.

88. Carl Rove, conservative political strategist, eroded John Kerry's credibility by attacking not his weaknesses but his strengths during the United States presidential election of 2004.

89. BMA resistance delayed implementation of the 'National Health Service Act' (1946) until 1948. The Minister, Aneurin Bevan, said that to overcome the doctors' reluctance he had 'stuffed their mouths with gold'.

90. Charles Stewart Parnell (1846-1891). Leader of the Irish Parliamentary Party, fell foul of the Bishops over his liaison with (married) Kitty O'Shea – they said 'by his public misconduct he has utterly disqualified himself'.

91. Muhammad, wishing to preach from the mountain, commanded that it should come to him. It did not move. 'If the mountain will not come to Muhammad, Muhammad must go to the mountain'. Francis Bacon Essays. 1625.

92. Browne, Noël. *Against the Tide*. Dublin: Gill and Macmillan, 1986. pp. 157-162.

93. The *Ne Temere* Papal decree (1907) required that all children of mixed marriages be brought up as Catholics. Sheila Cloney of Fethard in the dioceses of Ferns, a Protestant with three daughters refused to comply. The case (1957) became an international sensation with a local boycott of Protestant businesses organised by the Catholic clergy led by James Staunton, Bishop of Ferns.

94. DNA was described by Watson and Crick, Cambridge, 1953. Nobel Prize, 1962.

95. William Bligh, captain of the mutinous *Bounty*, 1789.

96. Opus Dei, founded 1928. Spanish right wing Catholic movement. In boarding school the author was regaled with Opus Dei readings during mealtime.

97. National Archive, TSCH/3/514997 C. This file contains a copy of the booklet.

98. The precise term used in Whyte, J.H. *Church and State in Modern Ireland: 1923-1970*. Dublin: Gill and Macmillan, 1971, p. 218.

99. By way of a slight digression and in the interest of balance the writer is not suggesting that this obsequious manoeuvre was by any means confined to Ireland. Latter day worshipers, who believe in Manchester United Football Club and no other God, should be reminded that Sir Matt Busby, the creator of their Deity, was known on occasion, when one of Their Lordships favoured Old Trafford, to drop to his knee on the touchline and kiss the ring. Sir Matt, however, great though he was, was bending the knee on behalf of something less than the electorate of a sovereign Republic.

100. A Grand Multipara, today, is a woman who carries 5 or more pregnancies beyond 20 weeks. The term was variably defined and in 1950 in Ireland the accolade required 10 pregnancies.

101. McCourt, Frank. *Angela's Ashes*. New York: Scribner, 1996. A description of urban misery and deprivation not received with universal acclaim by the citizens of his native Limerick.

102. Monsignor Frank Cremin, native of Kenmare, County Kerry, Professor of Moral Theology, St Patrick's Seminary, Maynooth.

103. With regard to dissenting clergy the case of Fr. Gerard McGinnity deserves honourable mention. As Dean at the seminary in Maynooth he courageously reported to the Bishops (1983) the inappropriate sexual behaviour towards male students of Michael Ledwith. McGinnity was victimised and rusticated to the West. Ledwith prospered and became President of the College. In close to 25 years, since Browne had consulted Cremin, little had changed.

104. Shakespeare, *Merchant of Venice*, Gratiano, Act 1, Scene 1.

105. During a visit to the Commonwealth Conference in Canada in 1948, Costello surprised everyone with his announcement that Ireland would leave the British Commonwealth and become a Republic. He had not been 'out' in 1916 nor against the Black and Tans, but in 1948 he stole the clothes of those who had been.

106. Fanning, Ronan. *Independent Ireland.* Dublin: Helicon, 1983, p. 166.

107. McCullagh, David. *The Reluctant Taoiseach: A Biography of John A. Costello.* Dublin: Gill and MacMillan, 2010.

108. The weaker vessel. St Paul to the Ephesians, 5:22-23.

109. Frank Colton, steroid chemist at the University of Chicago is regarded as father of the oral contraceptive pill (OCP). In 1951 he moved to the drug company Searle to produce Enovid, the first OCP.

110. Enovid was released in 1956 for 'menstrual regulation' but not until 1960 for contraception. The delay reflected the US Food and Drugs Administration's hypersensitivity following the Thalidomide (1957) disaster. After this time Irish Catholic women did not immediately embrace contraception. They did, however, develop a remarkable requirement, particularly at the more urbane end of society, for 'menstrual regulation'!

111. Boll, Heinrich. *Irish Journal (Irisches Tagebuch).* Published in German 1957. Republished, New York: Melville House, 2011.

112. Pejorative American jargon for public spending by a politician on local projects to earn the votes of his constituents.

113. A formal official Papal document with a lead seal for authentication. From the Latin *bulla* meaning (the lead) blister.

114. Vatican daily newspaper published since 1861.

115. Such a cross (although erected later, in 1976) on the Summit of Carrantoohil mountain was cut down by militant atheist vandals in November 2014. It was re-erected by local people within two weeks.

116. A plenary indulgence absolved the sinner of the temporal punishment for his transgressions. Their abuse was reminiscent of that to which Luther had objected.

117. The Papal Bull, *Decet Romanum Pontificem* (1521), by which Pope Leo X excommunicated Luther. Luther burned it publicly in Wittenberg.

118. 'To work is to pray'. The words were emblazoned on the wall of the author's boarding school study hall.

119. James Everett, National Labour Party, was Minister for Posts and Telegraphs. Everett was probably more concerned at this time (1950) about 'the Battle of Baltinglass', a controversy surrounding his parish

pump appointment of a crony to Baltinglass Post Office, than about stamps and statues.

120. William Wordsworth, English poet, 1770-1850. Poem 'The Rainbow'.

121. Spellman visited Clonegal, County Carlow, the putative home of his ancestors.

122. Summers, Anthony. *Official and Confidential: The Secret Life of J. Edgar Hoover*. New York: G.P. Putnam Sons, 1993, p. 167. Summers deals extensively with Spellman's activities.

123. Peter Sutherland, *The Irish Times*, 5 December 2015.

124. Dublin Diocesan Archive. 31.1.1954. XVIII/23/13/7.

125. Movie, *Divorce Italian Style*, 1961, made divorce a subject for comedy rather than hellfire and damnation.

126. Index Librorum Prohibitorum, a list of books Catholics were forbidden to read – often because of lascivious content. The prohibition was widely trumpeted in schools at this time.

127. Cross, Eric. *The Tailor and Ansty*. 1942, Republished, Cork, Mercier Press, 1995. Overt barnyard sexual dialogue offended the clergy who sent a deputation to burn a copy of the book in the subject's house.

128. Luke 8:11. The Pharisee stood apart and prayed, thank God I am not as the rest of men.

129. Hounds of god, a term applied to the Holy (Spanish) Inquisition. Sabatini, Rafael. *The Hounds of God*. 1928. Republished, House of Stratus, Cornwall, 2001.

130. Shakespeare, *Macbeth*. Act 3, Scene 4. 'I am in blood stepped in so far that should I wade no more, returning were as tedious a go o'er'.

131. 'Squares and crescents'. Ironic reference to private consulting rooms of important medical consultants in Georgian areas of Dublin. This reference appeared in a black propaganda flyer, illicitly circulated in working class areas, in order to undermine opposition to the Mother and Child Scheme. The IMA employed a private detective who allegedly traced it to The Department of Health. Noël Browne denied responsibility – he would, wouldn't he!

132. Harold Macmillan (1894-1986). Quaint patrician British Prime Minister, when asked what might derail a Government is reputed to have replied, 'Events dear boy, events'.

133. George Bernard Shaw, Irish playwright (1856-1950), was remarkably prescient regarding the future science of Immunology. *The Doctor's Dilemma* (1913). ' There is at bottom only one treatment for all diseases and that is stimulate the phagocytes'.

134. Liam Cosgrave, Fine Gael Taoiseach (1974), in an episode transcending normal levels of parliamentary farce, crossed the floor of the House to vote with the opposition against his own Government's Bill to introduce (a minimal) liberalisation of the law on contraception.

135. Rudyard Kipling, (1865-1936), British Empire poet, *The Ballad of East and West* (1889). 'When two strong men stand face to face, though they come from the ends of the earth'.

136. *Pax Romana*. A period of peace and stability in the Roman Empire consequent on strong central government, 27BC to 180AD.

137. John Milton, English Puritan poet (1608-1674). *Paradise Lost.*

138. Augustus Pugin, British architect, 1812-1852. Designed the British House of Parliament, St Patricks College Maynooth and also St Aidan's Cathedral, Enniscorthy – the seat of the Bishop of Ferns!

139. Shakespeare, *Macbeth*, Act 3, Scene 1.

140. Heller, Joseph. *Catch-22*. New York: Simon and Schuster, 1961.

141. Wimbledon, 1981, versus Tom Gullikson.

142. Urbane mandarin master of equivocation and obfuscation in BBC television comedy, *Yes Minister.*

143. Casey, P. Cullen, K. Duignan, J. *Irish Doctors in the First World War.* Dublin: Irish Academic Press, 2015.

144. Saints Cosmas and Damian, twin brothers, physicians and early Christian martyrs, 287 AD.

145. Rev John Rea, President of St Colman's College Fermoy (Catholic Diosescean Seminary for Cloyne), was a frequent contributor to the Cork branch of the Guild of St Luke, Cosmas and Damian. Cork City and County Archive, IECCCA/U689.

146. 'Polio resurgence in Pakistan following backlash from CIA vaccination ruse in hunt for Osama Bin Laden', Michael Edwards, ABC Web, 2014.

147. Many Irish specialist doctors, trained to a high level abroad, return to frustration in poorly managed under-resourced institutions. This, as much as anything to do with salaries, has been a source of malaise and recruitment problems in the system.

148. *Bodhaire Uí Laoighoire*. Irish Language idiom. A selective deafness which filters out that which it is inconvenient to hear.

149. United Nations World Population Prospects: 2011.

150. Maternal mortality: Fact sheet N°348. *World Health Organization,* June 2014.

151. Whyte, J.H. *Church and State in Modern Ireland: 1923-1970.* Dublin:

Gill and Macmillan, 1971, pp. 199-200. If de Valera had briefed the incoming Taoiseach, as would be normal, on the Hierarchy's objections, the whole disaster might have been avoided. A convenient oversight!

152. Luke 8: 2.

153. For example, the Hierarchy had objected to and prevented the application in Ireland of the early British National Health Insurance Act 1911 which would have benefited poor urban workers but not the landed classes. Barrington Ruth. *Health Medicine and Politics in Ireland 1900-1970.* Institute of Public Administration, Dublin, 1987, p. 49.

154. Health did not become a freestanding department until January 1947 with James Ryan as Minister. Before that it was part of the Department of Local Government.

155. Cooney, John. *John Charles McQuaid: Ruler of Catholic Ireland.* Dublin: O'Brien Press, 2003, p. 431.

156. Grande écoles. Elite French educational institutions above the common run of universities. St Patrick's College, Maynooth, would have considered itself more exalted than various other seminaries in Ireland which were producing mainly for the missions rather than the parishes of Ireland.

157. Donogh O Malley (1921-1968).

158. Galbraith, J. K. *The Affluent Society.* University of Michigan, 1958. Galbraith lampooned the divergence of standards in public and private facilities and amenities leading to suburban luxury and inner city decay. American medicine was moving in the same direction.

159. Matthew 11:19. 'The Son of Man came eating and drinking, and they say, "Look at him! A glutton and a drunkard, a friend of tax collectors and sinners!"'

160. Padraic Colum (1881-1972). Poem. 'The old woman of the roads.' 'O to have a little house! To own the hearth and stool and all! The heaped up sods against the fire, The pile of turf against the wall!'

161. Fergusson, Niall. *The Ascent of Money: A Financial History of the World.* London: Penguin, 2008, p. 234.

162. Robert Browning. English poet (1812-1889). *Pippa Passes* (1841).

163. Speaking of Taoiseach Enda Kenny on July 20, 2011, the *Guardian* reported, 'Ireland's prime minister has launched an unprecedented attack on the Vatican, accusing it of downplaying the rape and torture of Irish children by clerical sex abusers'.

164. Ashurst, Military Road. Killiney. McQuaid renamed it 'Notre Dame des Bois' – our lady of the woods. *The Irish Times* 12-2-2015.

165. *The Irish Times*. 12-2-2015.

166. The Local Appointments Commission was created by the Cosgrave Government after independence to counter improper influence in job interviews for the public service. It is now called the Public Appointments Service.

167. Irish Constitution (Bunreacht na hEireann) Article 44: 2,3. 'Every religious denomination shall have the right to manage its own affairs'.

168. Shakespeare, *The Merchant of Venice*, Act 1, Scene 3, Antonio, 'The devil can cite scripture for his purpose'.

169. Wilde, dying in Paris in 1900. 'The wallpaper is terrible, one of us will have to go'.

170. More than 150 Workhouses were built in Ireland under The Poor Law Amendment Act, 1834. Some remain as District Hospitals. In addition, St James', Dublin, St Finbarr's, Cork and Naas General are examples of such sites.

171. 40 million euro, at a time of national economic meltdown, was spent by the National Paediatric Hospital Development Board in a forlorn attempt to use the Mater Hospital site, *The Irish Times*, 14-8-2014. The product of their deliberations was an incongruous monstrosity, predictably rejected by town planners. The site available at St James', although constrained, is three times larger than that proposed at the Mater, *The Irish Times*, 5-9-2014.

172. Matthew 19:14. Jesus said, 'suffer the little children to come unto me'.

173. Galileo Galilei, Italian astronomer (1564-1642).

174. 1970s management jargon for unconventional thinking.

175. Nicolaus Copernicus, Polish, 1473-1543.

176. The tomb was discovered and opened by Howard Carter in 1922. He and others associated with the discovery died mysteriously giving rise to the superstition which is now recognised as having no scientific foundation.

177. Hensey, B., *The Health Services of Modern Ireland.* Dublin: Institute of Public Administration, 1988, p. 33.

178. Cooney, John. *John Charles McQuaid: Ruler of Catholic Ireland.* Dublin: O'Brien Press, 2003. 'Red Hat intrigues', pp. 232-233.

179. McNamara, Brinsley. *Valley of the Squinting Windows.* Dublin: Maunsell and Co, 1918.

180. The Health Information and Quality Authority (HIQUA) is the Irish Statutory healthcare watchdog body (2007). It is required by law to inspect all public but not private hospitals (at the time of writing).

181. Mount Carmel private hospital, Dublin, closed in 2014 amid much protestation. It contained the last Irish private obstetrical unit.

182. William Withering, *An Account of the Foxglove and some of its Medical Uses*, Birmingham, England, 1785.

183. Ernest Blythe (1889-1975). As Irish Minister for Finance in 1924, with the State strapped for cash he reduced the old age pension from 10 to 9 shillings per week. He was never forgiven by the people and became an electoral liability.

184. Australian Institute of Health and Welfare (AIHW) 2010-2011.

185. *The Irish Times*, November 12, 2013.

186. Testifying before the Oireachtas Health committee in December 2015, Tony O'Brien, Director General of the Health Services Executive used the term 'show trial'. He advocated a non-adversarial approach to provide redress. irishmedicalnegligence.ie. 23 December 2015.

187. Cooney, John. *John Charles McQuaid: Ruler of Catholic Ireland*. Dublin: O'Brien Press, 2003, p. 252.

188. Characters in *Gone with the Wind*, epic American Civil War film, 1940, based on novel by Margaret Mitchell.

189. A musical film, *The King and I*, 1956, based on Rodgers and Hammerstein composition.

190. Black, J.W., Crowther, A.F., Shanks, R.G., Smith, L.H., Dornhorst, A.C. (1964). 'A new adrenergic beta receptor antagonist'. *The Lancet* 283 (7342): 1080–1081.

191. Goldacre, Ben. *Bad Pharma: How drug companies mislead doctors and harm patients*. London: Harper Collins, 2012.

192. Mylan Cimetidine launch helps 'Street' regain stomach for generics; stock closes up over 20 per cent: Pfizer and SB move up with moves into disease management. Pharma and Med Tech Business Intelligence, 11-7-1994.

193. Statistica: the statistics portal, 2013.

194. This author sent a paper, lamenting the financial and environmental extravagance of disposables in surgery, to a prominent surgical journal in which he had published many times. It was rejected. The pages of the journal were replete with advertising for the said disposables.

195. In 2015 the Blackrock Clinic and other institutions are happy to advertise the limited opening hours of their emergency departments. Where do their clients go outside of these limited times?

196. EMTALA (Emergency Treatment and Labour Act), United States Congress, 1986.

197. Under 'Obamacare' new doctor-owned hospitals, a long-standing tradition in America, are banned. Already existing institutions are tolerated under a 'grandfather clause'.

198. Our Lady's Hospital for Sick Children (2013), resenting audit of how public money was being spent regarding the remuneration of its Chief Executive, said, 'The allowance is a private contractual arrangement between the Board and the Chief Executive'. 'On that basis, Our Lady's Children's Hospital Crumlin will not be making any public comment on the salary details of the private contract'. *The Irish Times*, November 18-11- 2013. It was, effectively, telling the State to mind its own business. In 2015, The Health Services Executive Director General found the finances of St Vincent's Hospital, Dublin impenetrable and intimated the possibility of 'special administration' for the institution. Tony O'Brien told the Dáil Public Accounts Committee that St Vincent's Private Hospital 'has a parasitic dependence on the adjacent State-funded public hospital'. *The Irish Times*, April 23-4, 2015.